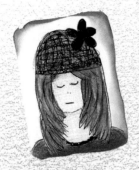

Marcia shares the intimate story of her own cancer adventure with words of peace, encouragement and humor. She continued to write, journal and cartoon through chemo, radiation, surgery and neuropathy. She wanted more than anything for those who followed her on this journey to have a guide and friend in the trenches.

It's All About the Hair

Your Cancer Journey

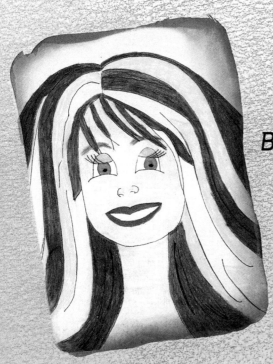

By:
Marcia McGee Ashford

DISCLAIMER:

   This book is written to help gals have a friend, a buddy, in the trenches on their cancer journey. It is not intended as a substitute for the medical advice of physicians. The reader should regularly consult a physician in matters relating to his/her health and particularly with respect to any symptoms that may require diagnosis or medical attention.

Dedicated to all the angels in my life!

On Earth
Family: Amber, Alex, Matt, Beverly, Uncle Ernest, Rowena
Girl Squad: Janice, Lynn, Jamie, Bonnie, Mechelle, Freda, Chris, Amelia, Lynn A, Jeanne, Becky, Jennifer, Beverly D, Lexi Grace

In Heaven
Randy, Mother, Daddy, Grandma Ashford, Poppie, Brooke, Katie Mae Burch, Papaw, and Mary Drake

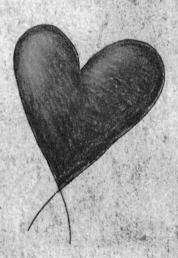

Introduction

February 8, the day that changed my life forever!
I was diagnosed with cancer. Yes, the Big C.

I asked to talk to someone with a positive cancer experience. I left the office with a prescription for anti-depressants and pain pills. I need support, not to be numbed out of my mind! Then was when I knew I had to do something positive to help myself and others with hurting hearts and a cancer diagnosis.

I understand grief and pain. My own personal journey over the past 10 years has been filled with it. Now I have cancer.

You wonder about the book title? Without hair who are we? Forget the cancer and focus on what's important, being bald! At first, that's the way it feels. The cancer is surreal. The hair is still real and on our heads!

Then we find out there is the ULTIMATE bad hair day! No hair at all! Every doctor warned me that the hair would fall out chemo #3 or 4. I planned in advance.

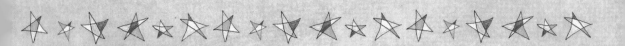

Wigs and caps started flying around. Everyone was trying to help me prepare for that moment when I was a bald headed woman. I still can't say it. Sounds like an oxymoron! Go ahead, try to say "bald headed woman" 5 times and keep a straight face! Then it finally happened. I survived. My head shines and surely glows in the dark.

This is a serious time in our lives. The goal of the book is to add humor, prayer, self reflection, and a sense of peace to lighten our journey. Most importantly remember that God is there with you all the time! "It's All About the Hair" is my version of Mark 16:15,

> "And he said unto them, Go ye into all the world, and preach the gospel to every creature."(KJV).

Seat belts fastened? Get ready to laugh, cry, vent and pray! Remember you are not alone, girlfriend! I am here, in the trenches, with you.

Bon Voyage!

Contents:

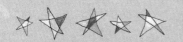 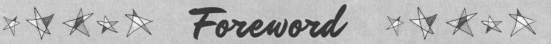

Foreword

"You MIGHT lose your hair or you might not", that is what I tell all my patients who are diagnosed with cancer and will be undergoing chemotherapy. As an oncologist I try to prepare my patients during their first appointment of what to expect over the next several months. Some of my patients come marching in the exam room prepared for battle with an entourage of family and friends armed and ready for warfare. Others come alone, either by choice or by necessity. Perhaps they are still processing or trying to carry the burden of the knowledge a little longer.   At some point, either initially or later during treatment, everyone, and I mean EVERYONE, is going to need help.

Marcia's book, It's All About the Hair, accurately portrays not only her fight, but the stages and experiences that many of my patients go through. She discusses the importance of family and friends during this time and the physical side effects and changes you might undergo during treatment. Chemotherapy reactions vary from patient to patient.   Some of my patient lose their hair, some don't. Some are sick day after day, week after week, others are only slightly nauseated. Some come in and say they didn't have the strength to take a shower, while a lucky few are able to ride their bikes to chemo. As an oncologist, I have seen patients on both ends of all spectrum. I encourage my patients to take advantage of the many resources and classes that are available. Knowing what to expect during each stage of treatment will help reduce some of the stress and possible side effects.

When patients learn they have cancer it is often all they think about. They wake up thinking about their diagnosis, and it's the last thing on their minds before they go to sleep. This worry only exacerbates stress and can elevate the physical side effects of treatment.

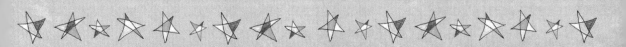

I try to tell my patients to stop worrying and to start praying. I try to explain to them the benefits of alleviating some of the stress by allowing others to help or to talk to their friends and family members about what they are going through. A good portion of my patients are not good verbal communicators. They internalize everything. For these patients, writing in a journal can help reduce some of their stress and free some of the emotions they are processing. Recent studies have shown that patients who wrote about their battle in a journal experienced fewer side effects and fewer unscheduled physician appointments. Another study published in The Oncologist, showed that writing for 20 minutes a day could have positive emotional effects for up to three weeks.

Two things never cease to amaze me – the power of faith and prayer and the unyielding strength of the human spirit. Combined I have seen these do amazing things. If you have been recently diagnosed with cancer, I encourage you to read Marcia's book and journal your experience. Once you are on your road to recovery, you might use your words and thoughts to help someone just beginning. There are going to be hard times, but you will be amazed at the care and love shown from others. Take their support and kindness and use it for strength.

Perhaps Marcia put it best when she said, "Stop and just breathe."

--John Waples, M.D.
Clinical Oncologist and Hematologist
Clearview Cancer Institute

Part 1:

Our Journey Begins

Diagnosis/Options

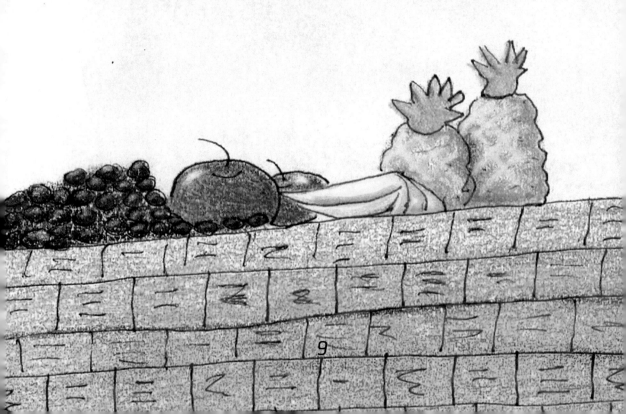

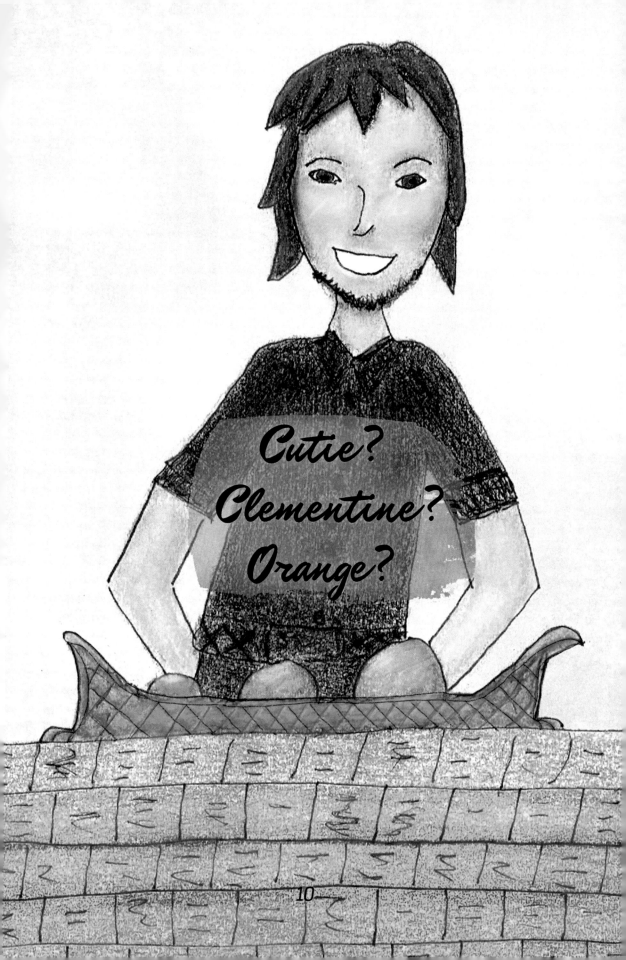

Suspicious or Naive?

Did you ever get the feeling something is wrong? You don't know what it is, have no evidence or proof but that inner voice is telling you something has changed and there has been a shift in your body.

Where do you go for help? A doctor? A friend or family member?

For several months I went from doctor to doctor. I had bronchitis, then pneumonia. I thought if I could breathe again all health issues would be solved.

My whole life my body had been good to me. Little did I know that now my immune system was fighting as hard as it could through 4 different rounds of antibiotics before the breast cancer was discovered.

Girlfriend, please understand your life is fixing to change drastically! You are going to have to be strong! You must learn a step at a time to ask questions, synthesize the answers, and be a fighter.
You can do this! I believe in you!

YOUR DISCOVERY STORY:

_____

_____

_____

_____

_____

_____

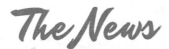

The News

Is there a single moment in your life you will always remember? You know exactly where you stood, what you wore, who was with you, even the smells in the air?

Being diagnosed with cancer is one of those moments! The world suddenly closes in on you. You can't think, breathe, or even stand. Your mind freezes to ease the pain.

Your first reaction is denial. The test results are a mistake. The tests have to belong to someone else......not you! Almost immediately your mind puts up a protective shield around others in your life. Your family and friends can't know this. If you tell them it will break their heart or worse they might blame you for contracting the disease.

How do you tell them? Who do you tell? First, it is your news and your body. Let me say that again! It is YOUR news and YOUR body.

You may want to share with just your immediate family for awhile. Enjoy their support and safety before spreading the news to others. You can share some of your story or tell them you don't want to or can't talk about it. It's up to you. You are in control.

You might ask a friend or family member to spread the word. Don't exhaust yourself by constantly repeating your diagnosis and sharing details. Save your energy for the journey.

HOW DO YOU FEEL ABOUT TELLING OTHERS?

There is no right or wrong way.
Just say it in a way that you feel comfortable.

_____

_____

_____

Size Really Does Matter

Cancer is cancer, no matter how large or small. No matter what type you have. After the ultrasound, the phone call I received said the tumor was small, about the size of a small, circular piece of candy. A lumpectomy should take care of the matter.

We went to see a surgeon for a second opinion. He said the tumor was huge! About the size of an orange. Looking back, I have to laugh. My son, Alex asked: "A clementine, a cutie, or a full-size orange?"

Guess size really does make a difference!

Who do you believe? What do you do? This invader has entered your body and it demands immediate attention.

Find professionals you feel you can trust and put together a plan to move forward!

Which reminds me! Don't forget to say THANK YOU to all the professionals you will meet on this new journey. They are there to help you!

WHAT SIZE IS YOURS?

_____

_____

_____

_____

Shopping Around for Treatments

Pick me! Pick me! This is bad. You need our services!

Have you ever felt so vulnerable? There is great fear... what should I do? How should I do it? If I get this wrong I could leave the planet!

Time and research are your best options! Read! Read! Read and research. Listen carefully to your options. Take a family member or friend to all appointments. Have someone take notes at every meeting.

Many times our family members are as stunned, or even more stunned, than we are. If they can't focus, have a close trusted friend do notes for you and your family.

Pray that you will be led to the right people. Let go and let God guide you. Don't be afraid to get a second or third opinion. It is your life!

If you know others who have had cancer, talk to them on a one to one basis. What treatments did they undergo? Where did they go for these treatments? Seeing others have survived should boost your confidence as well as giving you treatment suggestions.

WHAT ARE YOUR OPTIONS?
Compare your first and second opinions. Need a third one?

_____

_____

_____

The Chosen Plan

What have you and your family/friends decided? What choices are you going to make? Decisions have to be made. Treatments? Facility? Insurance coverage? Finances? What to do and where to go? Tough, life changing decisions.

All you want to do is go home and hide under the covers. Wake up and this dream will be gone!

Wake up! It's not a dream. Sadly it is time to be a grown up and accept what is happening in your life.

I send you hugs and prayers at this point. I remember seeing my family's faces. The surgeon talked to them in private then they came in to see me. Their sadness made my heart crack wide open!

There is a feeling of helplessness. Humiliation that you are some how to blame for contracting this disease. A feeling time is running out and you have to rush to a decision.

There is also the reality of money. You may not work and those co-pays add up quickly.

WHAT HAVE YOU AND YOUR FAMILY DECIDED TO DO FOR TREATMENT/ WHERE?

_____

_____

_____

_____

_____

_____

_____

_____

Have a Plan for Your Mental & Emotional Journey

What is it that keeps you on this planet? Makes you want to get up in the mornings? What gives you a sense that life is worth the effort?

You are going to have to find it, whatever it is. Is it God, your kids, your husband, a hobby, your parents, your job? Why do you want to stay here?

Dig deep and dig in because it is going to be a long journey!

Now, at the beginning of this journey, decide at least 2 things to keep you going. No matter how sick you are you can still do these 2 things for enjoyment and pleasure.

I chose writing and art. I wanted to help others who might go down the same path. I pray some of the things shared in this book will spare you some of the pain I had to go through on the way.

Are there things you started years ago and never finished? An old oil painting from school? Cross-stitch? A book? Pull them out and look them over. How about finishing a few things you started and never completed! Perfect timing!

You need things for quiet, you time. Things to fill time when family and friends aren't there.

You have to keep the ailing mind busy. Yes, the mind will be ailing too! What goes on in the body affects the mind!

IDEAS?

_____

_____

_____

_____

_____

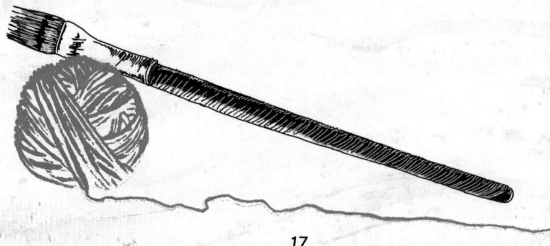

How Do I Get Through This?

ONE BITE AT A TIME

Beverly is my sister in law. She is kind, caring and wisdom pours from her lips. When I was diagnosed she summed up going through cancer treatments with the elephant story.

Imagine you are in Africa. There is no food except for one big elephant. You know you can't eat that elephant but you have to in order to survive. The thought of devouring such a creature is beyond your scope of imagination. What do you do?

You turn your back on the elephant and don't look at the whole thing. Instead you eat a small portion of it every time it's served. In the end the whole elephant will be gone and you will be finished. It will be over.

Is that not a wise analogy of the treatments we are going through right now? One small portion of it every time it's served makes it doable. Thank you, Beverly for breaking up a year of chemo, radiation, and surgery into one big, digestible elephant!

HOW DO YOU "STOMACH" THE JOURNEY?

How do you get from here safely and sanely to the other side?

_____

_____

_____

_____

Stop and Just Breathe #1

STOP! We all know what a stop sign really means. Come to a COMPLETE halt. Look both ways and then proceed. STOP does not mean come to a slow roll and race on to the highway! It means fully desist from movement.

Our minds are a whirlwind of activity and sometimes our worst enemy. Sometimes we can't shut it down to have a moment of peace. These pages are an opportunity to help you STOP the cyclone of thoughts and emotions even for a brief moment. It is a chance to regroup before you move forward on your journey.

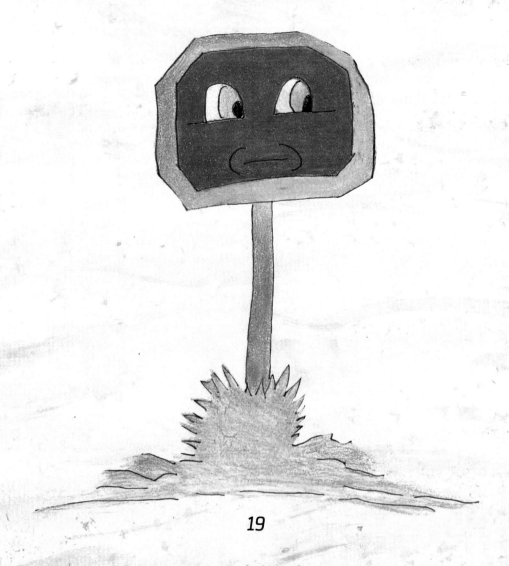

In a few short pages you have dealt with a cancer diagnosis, searched for treatment options, and committed yourself to getting well.

Congratulations!

Write about it. Draw. Play some relaxing music.
Let your mind go for awhile. Stop and release!

_____

_____

_____

_____

_____

_____

_____

_____

_____

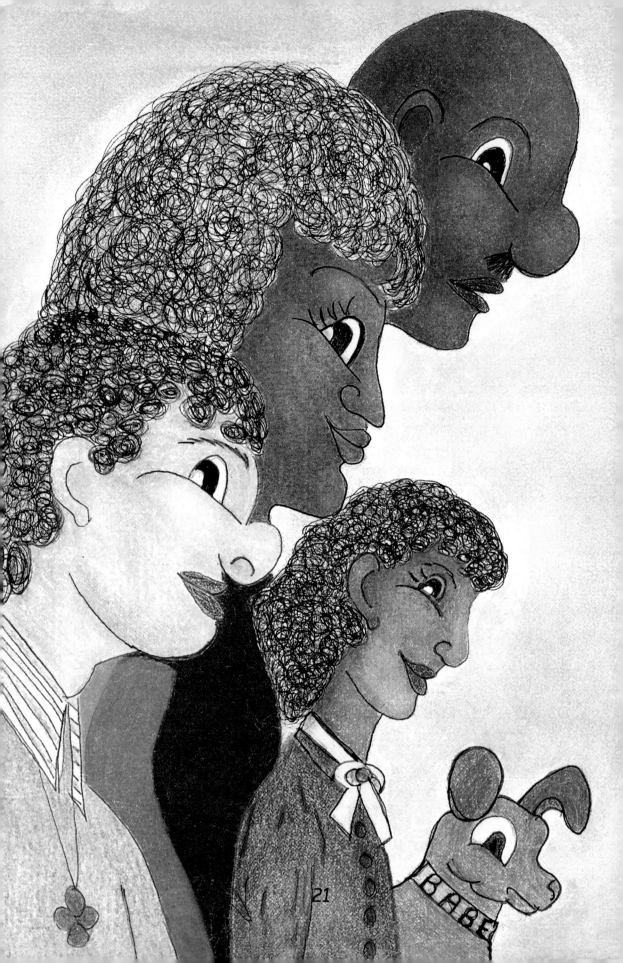

Part 2:

Family & Friends

Filling in the Blanks

Mother: _____ Father: _____

Step Parents: _____

Grandparents: _____

Brothers and Sisters: _____

Married: _____ Single: _____ Widowed: _____

Number of children: _____ girls _____ boys

Grandchildren/Great Grandchildren: _____

Best Friends: _____

Your Church / Sunday school class: _____

Co-workers: _____

Pets: _____

OTHERS YOU FEEL CLOSE TO, NOT MENTIONED ABOVE:

_____

_____

NOW: Look up! Look at this list! These are the people that love you! When you feel alone and depressed remember their names. Call them! You have "your people." You are not alone in this journey! They were in your life before the cancer and will be there during and after.

If you find yourself alone because of a recent move, divorce, change of job or other life circumstances feel free to reach out to support groups, churches, and community organizations.

You can create a new circle of relationships with individuals who will share the journey with you.

If you prefer to go this journey alone remember we are never truly alone because God is by our side always!

Cancer Requires a Team

You need to make a plan. Take a moment and put that thinking cap on. I KNOW how you feel. You do not want to be practical right now but realize that a few simple things done now can save you time and stress later on. You may go through chemo, surgery and/or radiation. That adds up to a lot of time!

Do you have a couple of changes of sheets? A barf pan? Lots of toilet paper and paper towels? Detergent? Plenty of underwear for quick changes?

Is your home handicap accessible? You might need a wheelchair (hopefully not) for awhile. Create a game plan now just in case.

Is there someone who could pay your bills if needed?
A power of attorney?

You will also need a personal support team. These will be individuals in your life you know you can count on. You have the list of all the people who love you and are on your side now go back and look at that list in a different way.

Who Can I Count On?

To drive me when I can't drive?
Pick up kids at school?
Take me grocery shopping or pick up things for me?
Lift heavy things-move things if needed?
Take care of dog/cat?
Household chores and mow the lawn?
Be your personal sitter if you require supervision because of treatment or surgery?
Reminds you that you are STILL the same beautiful person you were before the diagnosis?

No one to help? Ask the social worker at your doctor's office, a church or a neighbor. I bet you will be surprised how quickly they can find a driver, meal delivery, or other things you might need.

ADD YOUR PERSONAL NEEDS TO THE LIST:

1. _____

2. _____

3. _____

4. _____

For Gals with Small Children

How do you explain cancer to the little ones in your life? No matter how you tell them about your illness, they will still love you. Don't fret about doing it wrong.

IDEAS:

Keep it simple. Most younger children will be satisfied with terms like "sick", "it's a boo-boo", and "Mommy doesn't feel well."

If their daily routine will change have a game plan before talking to them. Kids find comfort in structure.

Have the discussion when they are rested and can be attentive. Don't do it alone - have a support system with you.

SOME COMFORT IDEAS FOR THEM ALONG THE JOURNEY:

A stuffed animal
A soft blankie
Start a small project, like a family puzzle, that brings you close
Hugs, hugs, hugs from their Momma

YOUR IDEAS:

_____

_____

_____

_____

Older Kids

Older kids are quite adaptable. They are very involved in their own social world at school, on the ball field, and in extracurricular activities. They have their own circle of friends who can help them get through your illness. Be sure they are allowed to stay in contact with this good support system on a regular basis. If you are too ill to take them places ask one of your trusted friends or family members to help see this is done.

They are also old enough to help you around the house. Do your older kids have assigned chores? If not, now would be a good time to start! They can do simple things. Dishes, trash, their own hair, washing and drying their own clothes, and making up beds are chores they can do to share the house and personal responsibilities.

We are all brought up in a reward world. We love stickers, gold stars, lollipops, and certificates. Make a job chart and stick it on your refrigerator door. Each chore accomplished earns them a sticker. Every week a new chart. They can keep their sticker charts and at the end of each month can turn them in to collect an even bigger reward.

You can decide what the BIG payoff is. You can have a big treasure chest ready right there at the house with extra treats inside or plan a picnic, short road trip, or the zoo! They will love it! They made the house look better, helped their Momma, and got rewarded for it!

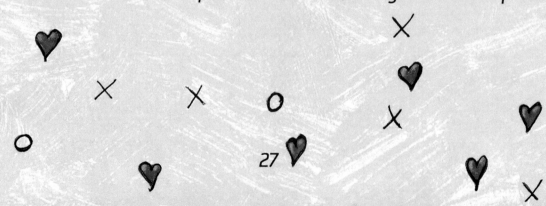

Good CAN come from our illness. I believe that! This is one area where you can see it happening. Your kids will blossom and grow as good stewards by practicing the first commandment, "Honour thy father and thy mother: that thy days may be long upon the land which the Lord thy God giveth thee." Exodus 20:12, (KJV).

BRAINSTORMING AREA!

Warning...construction going on! What can YOUR kids do to help YOU and to make them better stewards? Scribble, write, draw.

_____

_____

_____

_____

_____

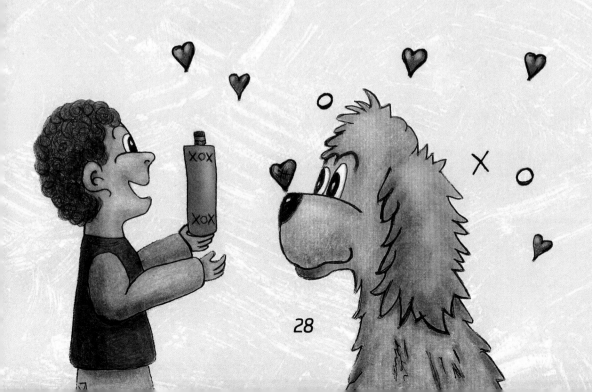

The Men in Our Life

So many times the men in our lives become second class citizens with our diagnosis. All your girlfriends and female family members are right there by your side to cry with you, encourage and keep your morale up.

What about the men in our life? The fathers? Husbands? Sons? What is happening in their lives right now? Who is by their side? I hate how men are supposed to be the strong ones. Men don't cry and all that other labeling. If the men in my life didn't cry when I was diagnosed with cancer I would think something was wrong.

Are the men in your life prepared for this whirlwind journey? No! You and I are not prepared so how can they "brace themselves" for the ride? Don't judge how a man behaves. If a man can't fix it he sometimes tries to lighten the mood by laughing it off. He is NOT trying to minimize your cancer; he is trying to cope in a way that is comfortable to him.

Avoidance is another common response. If I don't acknowledge it then the cancer doesn't exist. You and I tried that game too so understand he is buying time before accepting the reality of the situation. Our minds can only grasp so much at a time.

Is he angry? Yes! He let you down. Men have a natural protective instinct over the females in their life. He is trying to figure out how he let his guard down long enough for you to get cancer. I want you to know now he would do anything to take this cancer away. Our men would sacrifice themselves to spare us what is ahead!

Know the men in your life are NOT going to change a lot because of this. They are creatures of habit. They will gladly do what you ask to help but you will have to tell them how you are different, what you need from them, and remind them they are still loved by you.

The next page is for the guys you love so much. Give them the book. Let them read.

SUGGESTION:

You can give them a notebook/journal where they can record their own journey over the next few months. You have the book as your friend! Our men will also need a private place to weave through the ups and downs of what is ahead for all of you.

SOME HELPFUL IDEAS:
You might show the men in your life this list of ways to help on your journey. Feel free to add to this list, girlfriend!

• Take over day to day chores she can no longer do such as garbage, floors, dishes, laundry, etc

• Put a pan and peppermints beside the bed in case of night nausea

• A cold, wet washcloth works miracles when we don't feel well

• Fresh flowers on a bad day can do wonders beyond words

• Smile! Find laughter and share it with her

• The 3 most important words you can say "I love you!"

For The Men in Our Lives Only

The woman in your life has cancer. What do you do? You look her in the eyes, yes the eyes, and tell her she is beautiful! Make her feel like a girl. She will still be a girl, cancer or not if she knows she is attractive to you and that you still love her.

As the treatments continue you will no longer have your usual spouse/girlfriend. She may be replaced by a swollen faced, teary eyed, bald headed stranger. This stranger will demand plenty of attention because of her diagnosis. She will be clingy, sometimes distant, and always fearful of what is next. Remember this invader is costing her dignity, self esteem, parts of her body, and possibly more.

She is doing her best to be strong for you. She feels guilty because you have been tagged into her journey of cancer. She may be asking a lot of questions. What gave me cancer? Or she may be in the "why me" stage. What did I do to deserve cancer? What did I do wrong?

Cancer causes guilt. I'm sure you have it too. You can't blame yourself for her illness. It is not your fault! Life happens. I know you would gladly accept this disease for yourself if it meant she would be well. We women know that and appreciate your valor. But cancer doesn't work that way!

Our body has been turned into a pincushion and our skin may burn from treatments. It hurts! We are afraid of the future! We may be going through our hair falling out, our nails chipping off, eyebrows and eyelashes vanishing, our eyes swelling, tears that won't stop, our hearts breaking and a funny red rash on our faces.

One minute we are up. The next we are down. The chemicals swirling in our body and the disease put us on an emotional roller coaster. We are afraid we will disappoint you or leave you. We can recognize the danger of this path and accept it one step at a time.

WE:

1. Are tired and exhausted just dealing with the "Big C" diagnosis.
2. May be experiencing severe reactions to the treatment that is trying to make us well.
3. Can't eat. Can't even smell some things cooking during this time without nausea.
4. Cry in our sleep because that's the one time we let go of our pain.
5. Pretend to be stronger than we really are so you will not worry.
6. Want to still be your beautiful girl.
7. We love you beyond words.

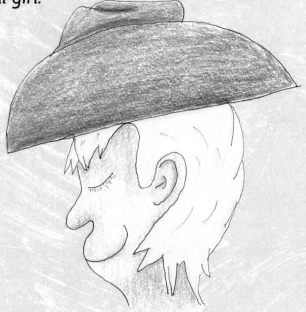

Thank you for STILL being in our lives! It takes strength and courage to share this journey!

Parents, Grandparents, and Siblings

You may find yourself regressing, falling backwards into a childlike state. That is okay! As a matter of fact, it is perfectly normal! You have a boo-boo and no matter how old we get we turn to our family to fix and mend what we can't. We know this is beyond their scope but still look to them for comfort and support.

Don't get upset when they put on the "happy" face for you. They are only trying to protect you by hiding how they really feel. Inside their heart is aching to see you with the Big C.

Have any of your family members been sick before? Remember how you put on the face for them? They are just returning the favor! Accept the disease for what it is and accept, with gratitude, the love that is headed your way. Many on this journey have already lost their parents and/or siblings so count your blessings!

No matter how much you tell them NOT to worry, they will worry anyway! Just understand, worrying is somehow a major part of love.

SUGGESTIONS FOR FAMILY MEMBERS:

• Remind her that this is temporary!
• Pray with her and for her.
• Let her whine but no permanent pity parties allowed.
• Don't quit loving because YOU can't stand to watch her suffer.
• Hugs may hurt - hug with caution!
• Keep a close eye on her as the treatments start adding up. There may come a time she literally cannot take care of herself.
• Remember someone may look good on the outside but cannot manage eating, drinking, or personal medications.

_____

_____

_____

_____

What Would My Family Do Without Me?

A cancer diagnosis is a wake up call. We suddenly see the world through a different pair of eyes. We feel vulnerable and mortal. Imagine our family without us? That's a tough one!

Cancer or not none of us are promised another day on the planet. Say "I love you" often to those you love! What can you do to make life easier for those you would leave behind?

I bought cards for each member of my family and close friends. I wrote a personalized note in each one, sealed them, and put them in a safety deposit box. Guess it's like having the last word!

My husband, Randy was killed in an accident so we never had that last goodbye. It hurts not to have that opportunity. I want my loved ones to have some sort of closure. I want to be able to say goodbye.

ARE THERE FAMILY TRADITIONS TO PASS ON?

Don't forget to include your secret eggnog recipe, Christmas traditions, and decade long honored rituals. Nothing is TOO small to add!

_____

_____

_____

_____

_____

_____

Heal old wounds. Say things while there is still time. Is there someone that needs to hear an apology from you? Is there anyone you need to forgive? Things you need to say while you still can?

Remember, we are healing our bodies and in the process our souls will change. Forgiveness and acceptance of others gives us a lighter heart.

_____

_____

_____

_____

I put important information in the safety deposit box such as bank account numbers, insurance policies, a copy of my social security card, and other miscellaneous data I thought would help if there ever came a time I could not speak for myself.

P.S. Had I known I would have put a lock of hair in my box. Too late!

Things We Don't Want to Talk About But Must Be Said

We do not need to add more grief to our loved ones' already heavy load! My friend Jeanne's father added her name to his checking account but not to his savings. When he became seriously ill she needed to purchase a wheelchair for him. She needed to take money out of his savings account.

Since her name was not on the savings account she had to hire an attorney to file paperwork so she, the daughter, could have the money to pay for the needed equipment. She ended up paying the attorney more than the wheelchair cost! Whew!

Just easier to get it done up front. Now!

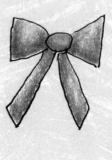

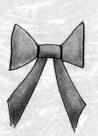
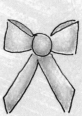

Get the Facts Organized!

1. Be sure you have the "someone else" you want on all of your checking, savings accounts, and safety deposit boxes.

2. Have you checked your beneficiaries lately? Your life insurance policy or retirement plan might need to be updated. Stocks?

3. If you have lost a spouse add a copy of their death certificate to the safety deposit box.

4. Medical power of attorney? Again, just in case you cannot speak for yourself? Who would it be? Ask before assigning, that is a tough one!

5. Discuss feeding tubes, living wills, comas, and DNR in a practical, realistic manner with the one chosen to guard your health.

CAN YOU THINK OF ANYTHING ELSE?

_____

_____

_____

_____

_____

_____

For Our Friends & Family

You are our support system. We love you beyond words. Love us for who we are right now. We are not the same person we were before diagnosis. It hurts and we are afraid of the future!

IMAGINE

Imagine someone putting you in long narrow tubes.
Injecting you with dyes, chemicals, radiation.
Imagine vomiting at the smell of bacon.

How would you feel? What would you do?

Don't say:
Poor thing!
Bless you baby!
Look how strong you are!
No words that will start the flow of tears for us.

We are trying to be brave for you.
We exaggerate how good we feel to make you feel better.

Those wigs and caps,
We have enough!
We smile when you bring us yet another one.
Why? Because we love you.

Do not judge us.
You do not know who you would be under the same circumstances.
We just want to be normal again!

Normal,
Able to be responsible for our own life, and
Not dependent on a chemical or treatment to save it!

Able to run and laugh,
Dance and cheer,
Able to feel the wind rush thru our hair.
Able to be alive!

Thank you for never giving up on us even in our weakest moment
Always by our side!

Doctor and Hospital Visits

FRIENDS AND FAMILY: YOU CAN HELP US GET ORGANIZED

When visiting doctors and clinics be sure you have all your bases covered. If you are organized when you walk in, it will make the initial paperwork easier for you and the office staff.

BE SURE TO BRING:

1. Your Driver's License or Legal ID
2. A second form of ID with a picture on it
3. Insurance card with policy numbers printed clearly
4. List of current medications with dosage (bring meds if you want)
5. Allergies to medications/foods/environmental
6. Dates and places of past serious illnesses and surgeries
7. Emergency contact names and phone numbers
8. List of questions and concerns to ask the doctor
9. Your family physician's name, number, and office address
10. A check, cash, or debit card to pay insurance deductibles

REMEMBER

Some medical and hospital bills will come in the mail, so have a special spot for those to be placed until you can deal with paying them.

Lynn's List

My friend, Lynn, put together a travel bag for me. You know the kind that can be taken to every doctor appointment, treatment, and day surgery. All disposable items are miniature in size making it easy for me to carry. She included things to keep me mentally organized, physically presentable, and emergency ready.
Thanks, Girlfriend!

THE LIST

Antibacterial soap
Barf bag, wipes, and gloves
Big envelope to store receipts
Chewing gum, cough drops
Contact holder and solution if needed
Cooling towel
Emergency twenty dollar bill/Checkbook/Debit Card
Eye drops
Ink pens, sharpie, pencils
Kleenex® - small pack
Notebook - with separate sections and pockets for each Doctor
Personal information packet: Include ALL info on previous page
Snack
Unscented lip gloss or ChapStick®
Ziploc® bags - different sizes
Change of clothes
Numbing cream for port if you are in chemo

Another Lynn Idea: have a small suitcase packed and waiting at the front door in case of emergency hospital visits!

Stop and Just Breathe #2

Whoa! How are you doing? We just talked about your team. You do not have to take this journey alone. Take a moment and think about you. How are YOU going to help YOU along this new life path?

OUCH! The reality that this life is only temporary has truly come forward in these last pages too. Remember to do what you can to make life easier for your loved ones if they are left behind. Get your house in order! Ask for help where needed.

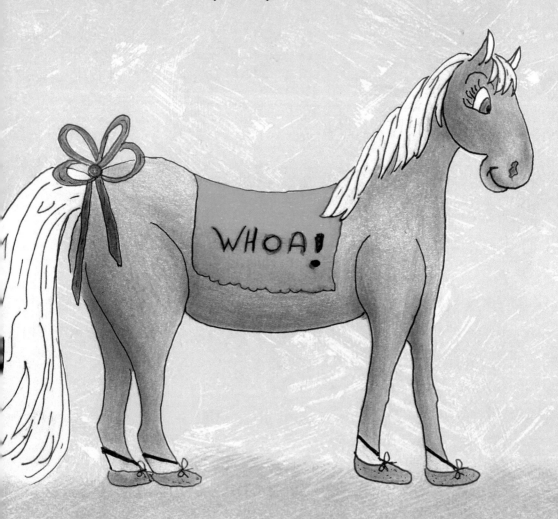

Take a moment for you. A moment to just breathe and regroup.
Write about it. Let your mind go for awhile. Stop and release!

_____

_____

_____

_____

_____

_____

_____

_____

_____

_____

_____

_____

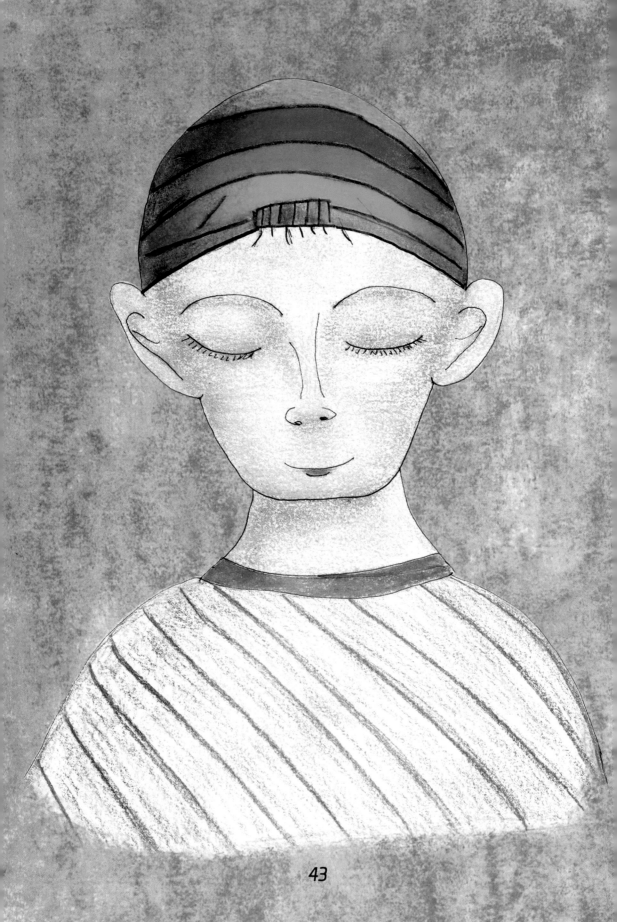

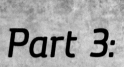

Part 3:

Physical Changes

Comfort is in Style

MAKEUP, JEWELRY, COPING, GIRL TIME!

It's tough right now. Your head is swirling with all the life changing information you have recently received. You look in the mirror and see that you are being replaced. It's like body snatchers are taking YOU away a piece at a time. If you are on chemo the hair is going or gone, the nails are turning dark and loosening and the nosebleeds. Oh, and don't forget the chemo tears that may stream down your red, swollen cheeks!

Every treatment you see a bit more of that person disappear from your psyche. You see your old charming self being peeled away layer by layer.

Clothes don't look the same. May be it's our posture, the port on our chest, marks on our body, the burning radiation places, the swelling of our face or the pain in our hearts but somehow those before cancer clothes just don't do it anymore.

I love dresses. They make me feel like a girl. That's why I need one on when I go to treatment. I need to be reminded I am still a girl. Course if I could, I would wear my puppy pajamas. How fun! Show up for treatment every week in a different pair of cute pajama pants!

End of chemo and post surgery suggestions – Anything you can physically put on your body! Cancer is cancer and there may come a time it cannot be disguised as anything else. No amount of makeup or a wig can make you look like you. Don't hide away in a closet! The days of your life are still ticking away. Go to the doc, the grocery, and get outside and breathe!

Remember this is just a phase you are passing through. Those cute clothes are still in the closet waiting for you to feel better!

P.S. If you are not experiencing any of these major side effects, YAY! Count your blessings!

What type clothing would be good for you and help you feel good about yourself? Is there a favorite color that could boost your mood?

_____

_____

_____

_____

_____

_____

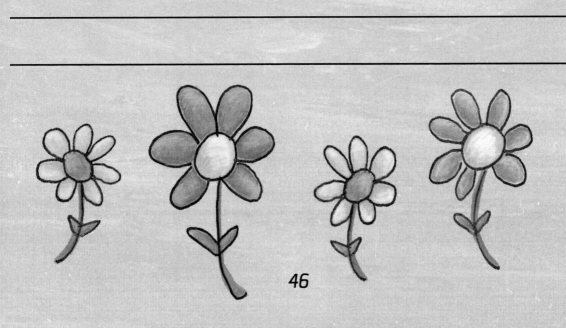

Rings and Other Obsolete Things

Think of all the jewelry that you have adorned your fingers and toes with in your lifetime. Beautiful, sparkling fun jewelry, and brilliant colors to accent your extremities.

Look at them. Take a good look at them because things are going to change. Change and disappear. I couldn't believe it, but there does come a time it's just not worth putting a lot of accessories on. Somehow I just can't get the same "put together" look.

Downsize the jewelry. A pair of earrings, and maybe a light weight bracelet are sometimes all my body can carry. Fingers swell so rings might not be a good idea. Necklaces are SO tough to do with a chemo port and who wants jewelry in radiation?

Purses, or totes, need to be small and practical or one big bag where you put everything. Don't forget to put on your favorite lipstick! No one can go without a spot of color!

Remember less is more on days when you are not feeling your best. It's not a fashion show. Be clean and comfortable.

I wore jewelry to port installation. I didn't know! No one said it wasn't a fashion show...ha. Oh and contacts! Sadly you can't wear them for surgery either. How do they expect us to see what is going on?

Of course I'm the gal who wants to invent "Glitter Port Covers". If we have to have ports they need to be tastefully covered in outfit coordinated colors and designs. Oh, and how about fake diamond studded radiation tattoos?

Makeup? Keep it light and simple. If you are doing chemo you might want to learn how to paint on false eyebrows. Did you know some people get their eyebrows tattooed before they start chemo?

Cool!

Remember it's ALL about the hair!

MAKE SUGGESTIONS TO DOWNSIZE YOUR MAKEUP AND ACCESSORIES:

_____

_____

_____

_____

_____

_____

_____

_____

_____

Eat Like a Pig and Wear a Wig

OR IS IT WEAR A WIG AND SWEAT LIKE A PIG?

In the introduction I talked about my first reactions to losing my hair. Funny looking wigs were flying around and everyone chimed in to try to cover my bald head. Amber works at a hair salon so all the girls were on board in this new adventure! There was an obsessive need to keep my head covered with hair EVEN if it had to be previously grown and worn on someone else's head or synthetically made.

Finally, my wig in tow I bravely faced the ultimate outcome. I was set for action.

What no one told me was that in one hundred degree weather you wear a wig and you sweat like a pig! I could picture myself fainting in the grocery store parking lot, the perfect wig still firmly planted on my head, but the rest of me in a big puddle.

The crocheted caps? Same! Hot and steamy! What is a girl to do? First off, postpone the sunbathing! We do not need to battle the heat midday with our artificial tresses. Save the sun surfing for next summer!

What an amazing thought! My head, and yours, have probably not seen this much sunshine since we were infants. Bald to the world is not the perfect fashion statement BUT it is the perfect setup for sunburns on a whole new part of you! Ouch!

My compromise? Short, brief jaunts out in the early morning hours and from sunset on. Fight the heat wisely. We are already rundown, dehydrated, and probably malnourished. Don't add to your discomfort by trying to do activities in the heat of the day that you could easily do another time.

Don't worry, if it's winter when you read this we will freeze! We will love our wigs and cute caps! A coat for our little bald heads!

How have you changed your daily schedule because of the weather and your ability to cope with it?

_____

_____

_____

_____

_____

_____

_____

_____

_____

How is the Real You?

WHAT PHYSICAL SIDE EFFECTS ARE YOU EXPERIENCING
FROM THE TREATMENTS? HOW DO YOU COPE?

_____

_____

_____

ARE YOU EATING? DRINKING PLENTY OF WATER?
FOLLOWING DOCTOR'S ORDERS?

_____

_____

WHAT ARE YOU DOING FOR YOUR EMOTIONAL HEART?
TO NURTURE YOUR SPIRIT?

_____

_____

HOW IS YOUR HAIR (OR LACK THEREOF) LOOKING TODAY?

_____

_____

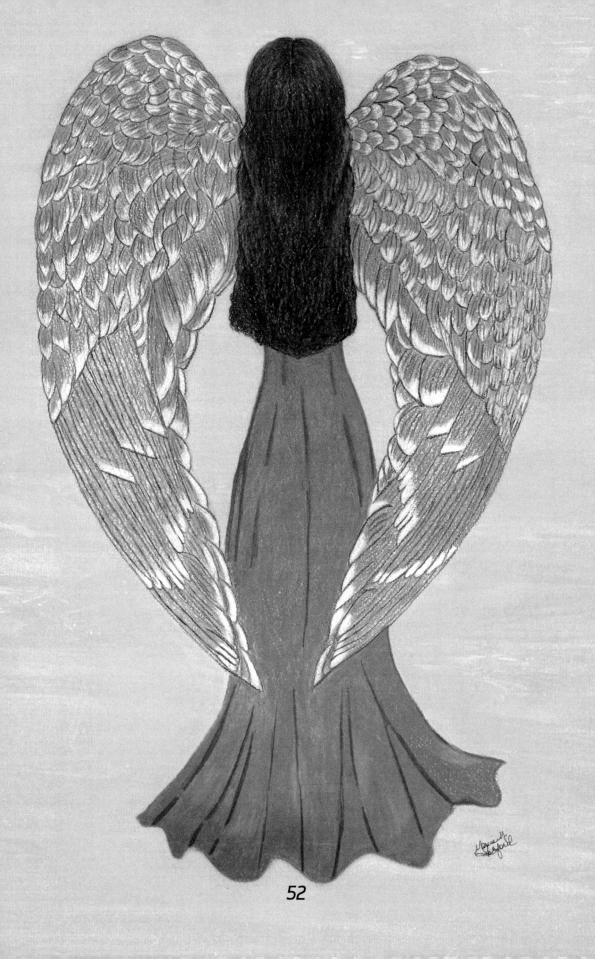

52

Stop and Just Breathe #3

You've Got Mail! We just talked about how your whole life is changing. Your lifestyle, wardrobe, makeup, jewelry, and the sense of losing control.

How does this REALLY make you feel? You are still the beautiful woman inside you have always been but the dramatic changes on the outside make you lose that image. Keep her, the real you, tucked deep in your heart.

Stay away from negative people. They can bring you down. You have to take care of you. Design this experience to get well physically and emotionally.

I bet you've nurtured everyone else and not yourself. We all want it all and to live every moment to its fullest. We push our limits. It's time to STOP IT. Stop what you are doing and examine your life.

Are you overextended at work? At home? Then it's time to ask for help. You are good at giving it, now receive it with gratitude. Let others do for you!

Take a moment for you. A moment to just breathe and regroup. Write about it. Draw. Let your mind go for a while.

Stop and release!

_____

_____

_____

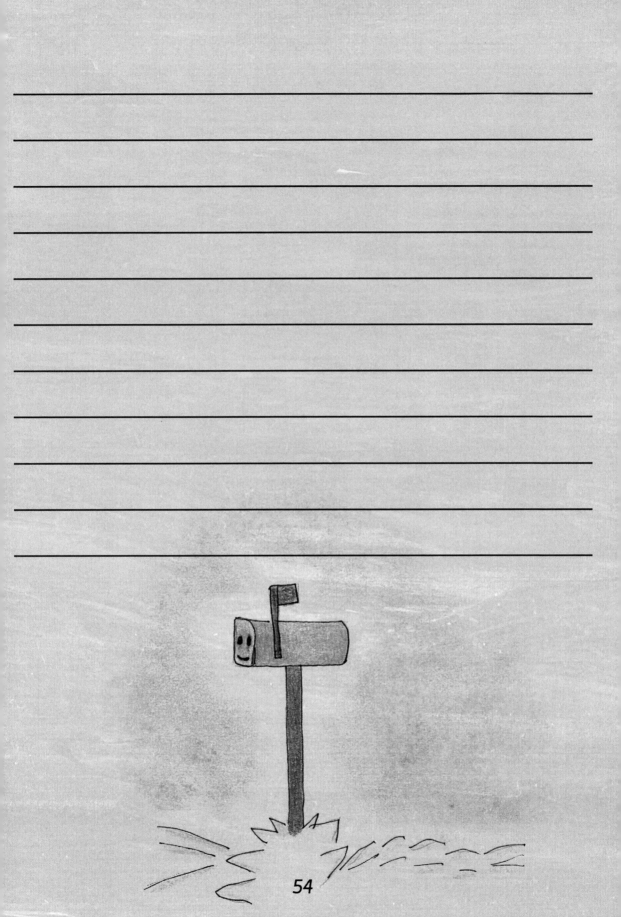

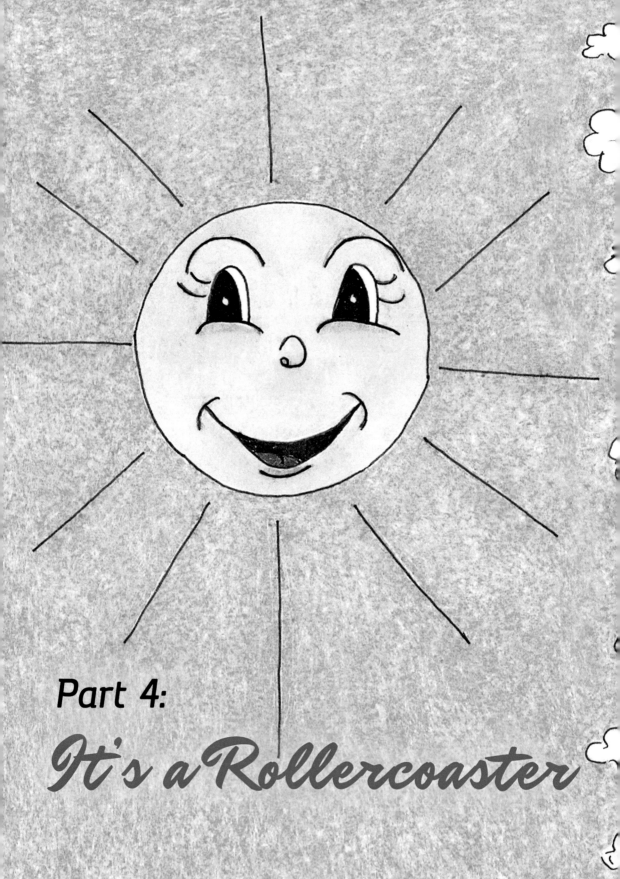

Part 4:

It's a Rollercoaster

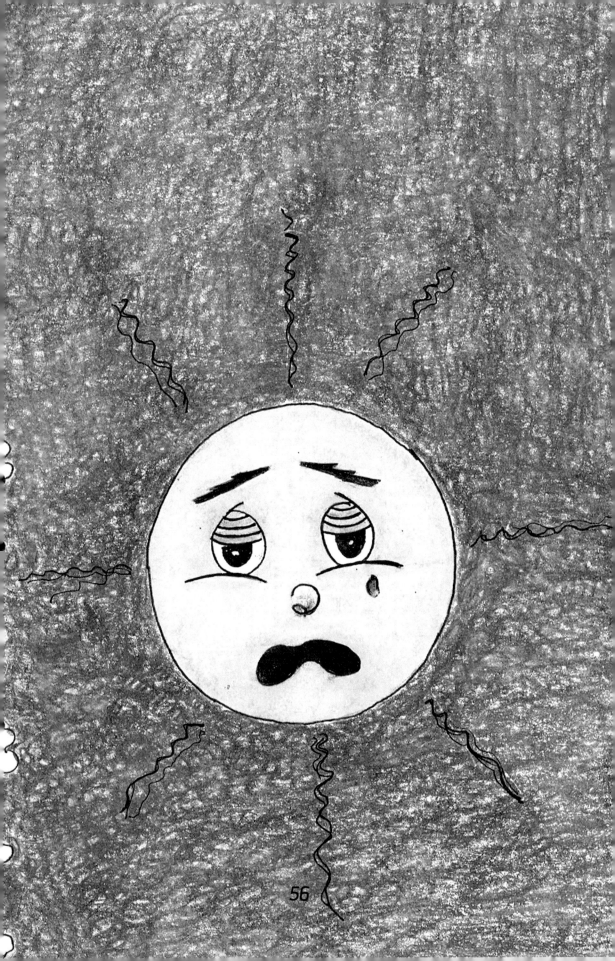

Riding the Ride

THE BLAME GAME

I know you are going through a lot right now. You have been diagnosed with the Big C and you are trying to figure out how you got here. There is a ton of guilt weighing you down!

My family and I were just talking. I am the one who eats healthy and tries to avoid things that make me sick. I balance my supplements, get plenty of sleep, and drink lots of water. So why am I the one with cancer? Again I ask the question "Why me?"

We start the blame game. What gave us cancer?

Plastic bottled waters?
Electrical current?
Soy?
Sugar?
Not enough fiber?
Too much sun?
Not enough sun?
None or all of the above?

The possible list is endless and gets us nowhere. We have to accept we have cancer. The why? That may be beyond our scope of knowledge.

Don't let guilt weigh you down! It is not your fault!

LET GO OF ANY GUILT YOU MIGHT FEEL!
We are women and we tend to hold on. Let it go here!

_____

_____

_____

_____

_____

_____

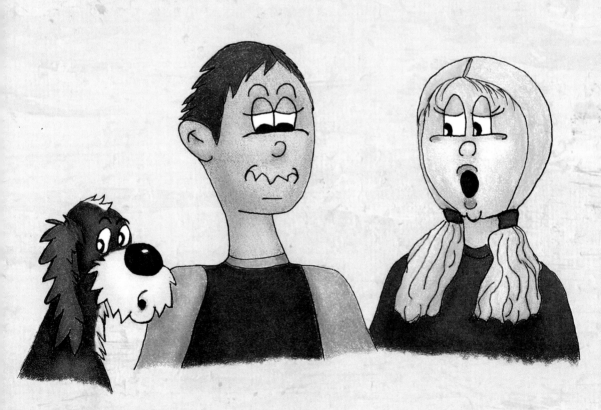

Anger

Women are taught to be ladies and we all know ladies don't get angry. Right? Wrong! Aren't there times you have so much rage it boils over and on to those you love? Don't you get angry sometimes?

Are you going through the pain of port installation, chemo, radiation and other treatments? You see others living a lifestyle that screams cancer or heart attack and yet you are the one here.

Are you angry yet? Now don't be nice, be *honest*. I repeat, are you **angry** yet? This is a safe place to vent. Don't hold back. Get the pain out of your heart! Write. Draw. This is your personal space. Release the anger demon!

_____

_____

_____

_____

_____

_____

_____

_____

Grief

We grieve for major life changes such as a cancer diagnosis. Is it natural to grieve for parts of your body? You bet it is! We came into this world a complete package, pure and unadulterated. Now you're losing bits and pieces. These pieces are a part of the complete you!

Grieve... grieve... grieve! It is okay! Cry, scream, write about it, draw it, tell a trusted friend. If you don't grieve it will wear a hole in your heart and the emotional pain will create physical pain. Get it out!

We grieve and move on. We find things to help our hearts heal along this journey. Writing this book is a major part of my healing. Reading this book and participating in the writing activities is, I pray, a part of your healing!

God didn't promise us to get to heaven without suffering and with all our parts! The important thing is to get there...even if it's piece by piece! Bet you think you deserve a break and ole' cancer pops into your life!

TELL YOUR STORY! GRIEVE, GIRLFRIEND! GET IT OUT!

_____

_____

_____

_____

Humility

Those of you who have birthed children know what a humbling experience it is. There is no privacy, no modesty, and no glamour. After hours of labor you pop out a goo covered baby and feel unimaginable pain.

They say after a few years the memory of that pain leaves us. I don't believe that. I believe it is always somewhere hidden inside. The joy of seeing our children grow just covers it up.

Cancer is a humbling disease. There are no designer ports, cute hospital gowns, or any privacy. I take chemo in a room with up to six other individuals. I look in their faces and I see a mirror of my own. Sadness. Loss. Nausea.

Will the pain inflicted on us during this time also sink deep in our souls and disappear? I hope so. Will we forget the day we barfed on the staff? Accidentally pulled the alarm? Peed in our pants when they stuck the needle in the port for the first time? Maybe!

WHAT HUMILIATING STORY DO YOU HAVE TO TELL?

_____

_____

_____

_____

_____

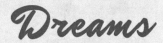

Dreams

What do you dream about at night? I am always on the farm riding my horse "Master". I feel like I am flying! Free! The wind rushes across my face, his mane tickles my nose and I laugh. Then I wake up.

My legs are heavy, my eyelids swollen almost shut. I look in the mirror to see real tears, not the chemo ones, stream down my face when I realize that image is me. There is no changing it. No wig or lipstick can cover the horror I see. Nothing to patch the hole in my bleeding soul.

I look at pictures made four short months ago and ask myself: "Where Did This Woman Go?"

Yawn! I can't change things so I go back to bed and continue to my precious dream! Giddy up!

WHERE DO YOUR DREAMS TAKE YOU?

_____

_____

_____

_____

_____

Sweet Dreams, my friend.

Want Some Whine With That Cheese?

Remember when the body hurts so does the spirit. Our souls are in a physical body so they are intimately intertwined.

Do you have days you can barely lift your head? You want to curl up in bed and stay asleep? You are too tired or too sick to face another morning?

If you answered yes to all of the above, you must be in chemo or radiation! Welcome aboard the drain train! Vomiting, diarrhea, a swollen face, and the inability to eat may have become part of your daily routine.

Your days may be spent walking between the bed and the bathroom. I've had days I could not even walk to the front door to answer the doorbell. Too much energy needed!

Major treatments or not, you may feel isolated and lonely. It is easy to feel alone on this journey. You are experiencing something that hopefully no one else in your immediate circle is. Doctors are interested in your physical condition. Family and friends satellite around you trying to keep day to day things as "normal" as possible.

Where do you go to release the pain in your heart? Whine! Whine! Whine! It's okay.

You can't be anything to ANYONE when you feel this way. You have to take care of you!

Sleep in your puppy pajamas all day. Watch all those old cry movies you never had time to watch. Cry! It's okay!

Remember this is only a temporary parking place. Rest.

YOUR TURN TO WHINE. GIRL LET IT OUT!

_____

_____

_____

_____

_____

_____

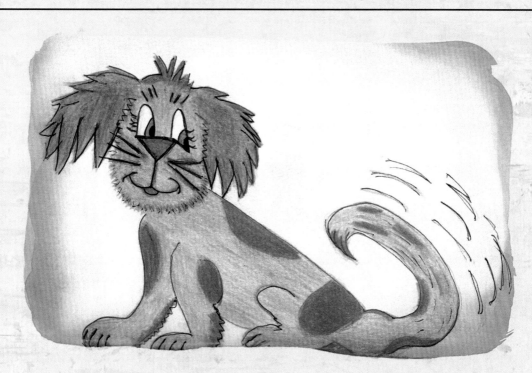

Humor

It's hard to find something to laugh about with a cancer diagnosis. Even the everyday things you would normally find joy in don't feel happy anymore because of your life changes.

How about some silly cancer treatment facts to get you started?

DID YOU KNOW:

1. Hair stops growing during chemo so the hair that DOESN'T fall out has no gray roots! You will be gray root free for chemo! What roots you have!

2. You save money by not buying shampoo, conditioner, and hair color.

3. You can eat anything you want or can stomach and not gain weight.

4. Have your friends take you to the other side of town to shop once you lose your hair! That way your home neighborhood does not see your cute, little bald head!

Hope you smiled! Humor is important in our situation. If you can laugh you can survive. Sometimes things that would normally not seem funny are hysterical. Maybe our bodies need that release to keep us healthy and alive.

Find some humor in your life today. Want to add to the silly cancer treatment list? Go for it! Laugh it's good for your health!

_____

_____

_____

_____

_____

_____

_____

_____

_____

_____

Are you feeling better? You know we can laugh at ourselves too. Lighten the moment.

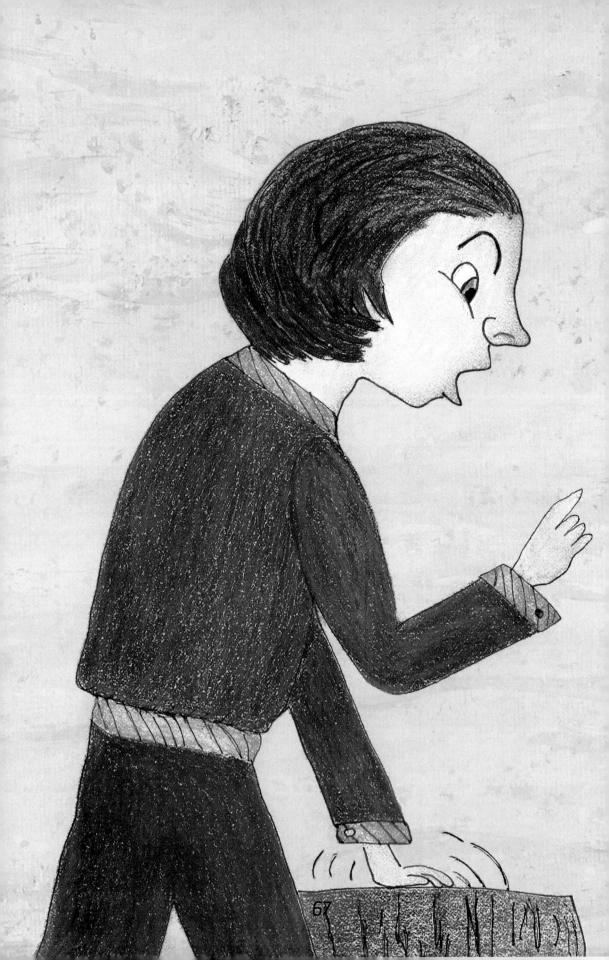

Stop and Just Breathe #4

Girl, have we released a lot of emotions! How are you doing? Is there something you need to rant and rave about? Did one of the journal entries stir up some old things in your life that need to be addressed? Here is your spot! Go for it!

Take a moment for you. A moment to just breathe and regroup. Write about it. Draw. Let your mind go for a while. Stop and release!

_____

_____

_____

_____

_____

_____

_____

_____

Part 5:
Reality Starts to Sink In

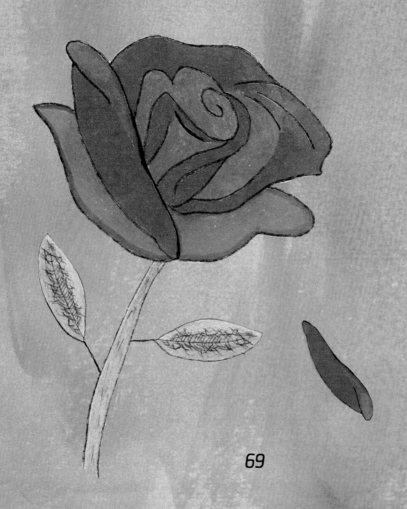

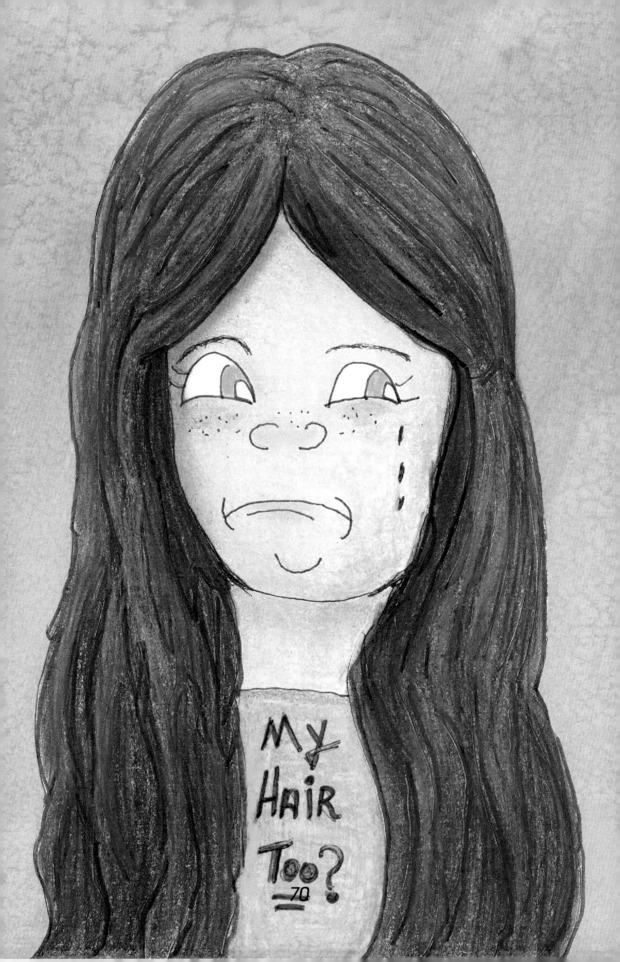

Checking in on You

Sometimes we are up! Sometimes we are down! How are you at this point of the journey?

A few weeks ago you knew very little about cancer, wigs, fake eyebrows, and side effects. Now you are experiencing them first hand. You have stepped outside your world into a "Twilight Zone" of pain and suffering you could never have imagined.

We women spend our lives trying to look our best. Haircuts, hair color, push up bras, the right clothes with the right fit, and of course, great nails. Suddenly you are thrown into a world of shedding, baldness, a bra hurts, clothes are only for modesty (not style), and the nails might fall off! When you go out no one even recognizes you!

You may look in the mirror and do not know that person. Puffy eyes, a rash on the cheeks, bleeding nose, and running eyes may stare back at you. You look your age. No 2x worse! You feel your age. No 4x worse! We don't mean to be shallow but we do know how we look has an effect on our emotions.

There is a strong need to see, touch, and hug those you love. You are comfortable when your nest surrounds you.

Your circle of friends may shrink. Remember you will have more free time now. They are still working and trying to pay the mortgage. They may not be available all the time.

Some may have a cancer phobia and can't deal with your illness. Don't judge them. They may need time to accept your diagnosis or they may have a valid reason they can't go on this part of the journey with you. Just let go. There will be others along the way to take their place.

JUST BETWEEN US HOW DO YOU _REALLY_ FEEL?

_____

_____

_____

_____

_____

_____

_____

_____

_____

_____

_____

_____

Social Activities

How do you have a social life? How do you continue with the activities that have always been so important to you?

Parties, church socials, highly seasoned food and noisy places may not be in the game plan. How can you enjoy a party when you have to go to the bathroom every five minutes? When everything you eat causes diarrhea and flatulence? When you have surgical stitches or radiation burns to protect?

The music is loud. People are talking over music so they are even louder. How do you cope with the extra noise? It sounds like screaming in your ears. Your brain is not processing what they say. You are not like them. You feel isolated, left out, alone. You are not the social person you were a few months, weeks, or even days ago.

It's okay. Your mind and body are on a different plane of reality. Our world is very small. It may consist of your family, church family, and the professionals who are taking care of you. There may be no energy to be a social butterfly right now.

One of my thrills is going to the hat basket every chemo and seeing the new hats ladies have crocheted. Talk about a wild and crazy social life!

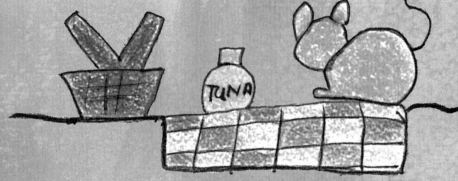

HOW HAS YOUR SOCIAL LIFE CHANGED?
I know, what social life?

_____

_____

_____

_____

_____

_____

_____

_____

Missing People? Give them a call! I bet they don't even know
they are missing from your life!

Hurts and Disappointments

We have all had more than our share of hurts and disappointments. It is how you handle them that makes a difference. We can wallow for years or after a reasonable amount of time start the job of shoveling ourselves out of the hole to stand back on solid ground.

How does one describe a "reasonable amount of time"? Good question. I have NO idea. I think it depends on the circumstances and the depth of pain you are experiencing.

I do know it is important to remember God is there for you. "Be careful for nothing; but in every thing by prayer and supplication with thanksgiving let your requests be made known unto God. And the peace of God, which passeth all understanding, shall keep your hearts and minds through Christ Jesus." Philippians 4:6-7, (KJV). God's peace, the peace that passes all understanding! What an amazing concept!

Does that keep you warm and fuzzy at night? What about when the 2 am nightmare wakes you up and you can't go back to sleep? Many of us are tactile people and need a tangible comfort item.

Mine is a huggie pillow. There are just times you just need to curl up in a fetal position and latch on to a big ball of fluff! There is something so comforting about the squishy way it shrinks as you hold it down and it puffs in your arms when you release pressure. You know exactly what I am talking about! Go ahead and smush it! Now don't you feel better?

How about a rocker? It wasn't that long ago all adults had rocking chairs and leisurely rocked their way into the early night hours sitting on the front porch with a steady, consistent and comforting rhythmic pattern. Think of the gentle rock back and forth. Slow and gentle, a consistent pattern to release the day.

You may have a special stuffed animal you had from childhood, won at a fair, or a friend gave you since you were diagnosed. Hug it! Hug away! It can't hug back at 2 am but you can wrap your arms around it, see its little face, and know you are not alone!

I have a confession to make. I wear my puppy pajamas and listen to Christmas music every time I write. It does not have to be Christmas to listen to the incredible music of the season. You can have Christmas all year long! Try it! It is guaranteed lift to your spirits!

There is a hurt child inside your adult, tender body. What can you do to create comforts your child-self needs right now?

_____

_____

_____

_____

_____

_____

You Have My Permission to Take a Break

It is important to take an occasional break from this illness. Do small things that you can manage. Go out for ice cream, a play date with your kids, a picnic with your family, or a date night. Get out of your own head for a while and have fun! Forget! Laugh!

Don't let this disease devour and define you. Remember you are still the same person you were before your diagnosis. You just have to get through this phase of your life and disease.

Have you ever met someone that only talked about their illness? They own it! They bought the disease and claim it as theirs!

Don't own cancer! It is a temporary place to be. See past this disease and into your cancer free future.

I Corinthians 6:19, "What? know ye not that your body is the temple of the Holy Ghost which is in you, which ye have of God, and ye are not your own?"(KJV). I am grateful to be a temple of the Lord. Doesn't that put everything into a different perspective for you and me?

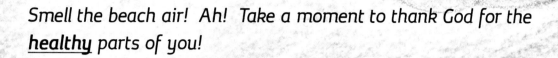

Smell the beach air! Ah! Take a moment to thank God for the **healthy** *parts of you!*

_____

_____

_____

_____

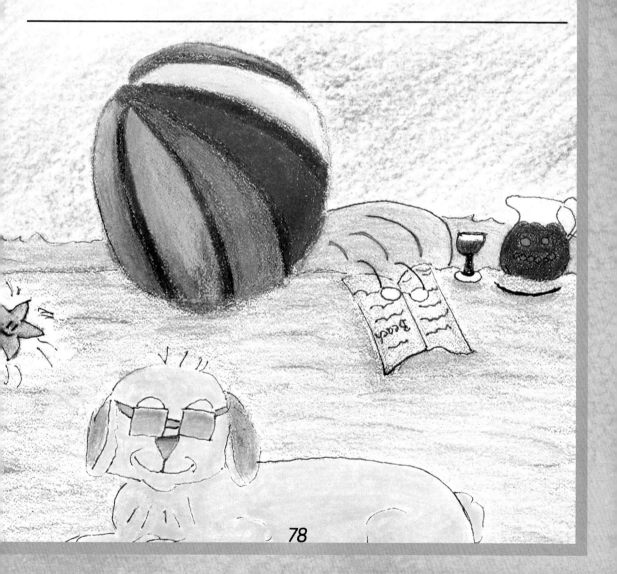

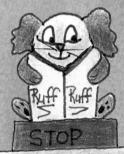

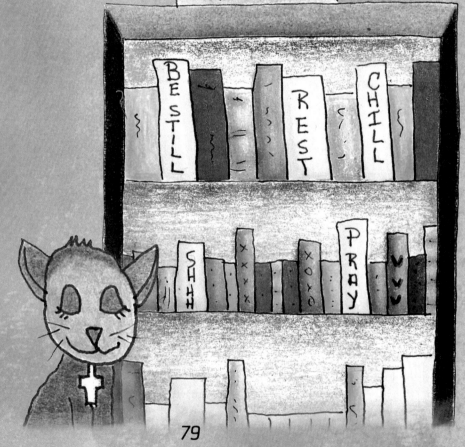

Stop and Just Breathe #5

Shh! That's what we tell children when we go to the library or just need our quiet time. Now I'm asking you to sh-h-h from the noise of the world a minute. Put on some quiet music if you like. Sit alone.

Stop and release what is on your heart today.

_____

_____

_____

_____

_____

_____

_____

_____

_____

_____

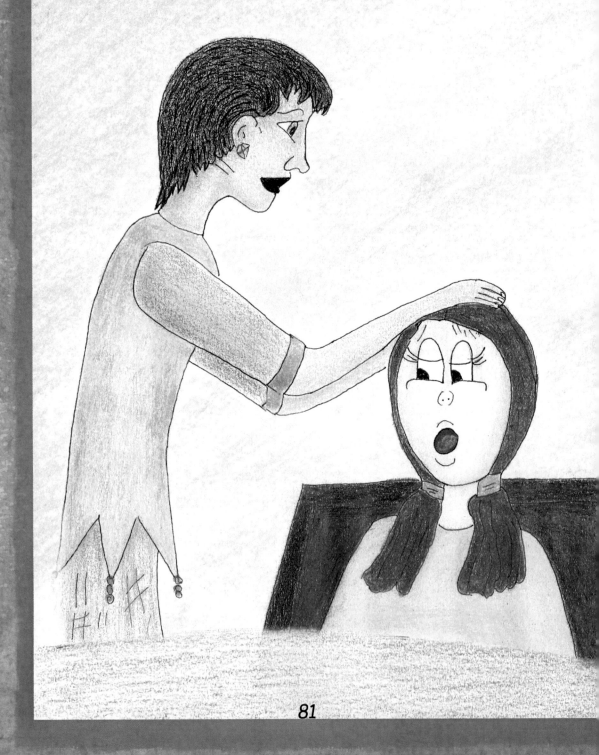

Part 6:

It's All About the Hair

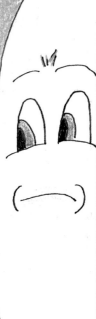

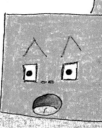

It's All About the Hair

What makes you feel feminine? Your hair flowing beautifully around your face? Your dress curving to your figure? Your long, well manicured nails? When cancer strikes many of the things that make us feel girlish may disappear. It leaves us feeling more like an "it" than a woman.

Who are you without your hair? I still have melt downs. I want to be normal. To blend in. Outsiders see you in a wig or a cute hat they know you are "one of them." Horrible! To be labeled one of "those" cancer people.

I let my hair grow for three years. I was so proud of it. Finally, it was long. Healthy and beautiful! Then came the diagnosis. It's cancer... and by the way, your hair will fall out the third or fourth chemo treatment.

My hair? My beloved hair? The hair I lovingly washed and combed every morning. The hair that had consistent root touch-ups to keep the red in and the gray away.

Amber, my daughter, always did my root touch up. The first touch up after I was diagnosed she said, "How about I cut your hair to your shoulders? You know it's going to fall out eventually". I thought I was going to barf on the floor.

The morning after the third chemo I couldn't even get a comb thru my hair. It was like it melted in one big wad. Amber could not even separate the mats. She got her friend Shelby to help. She said, "Imagine you are detangling a dog. Take it one tiny mat at a time." They both worked for at least an hour detangling my mess.

Shelby put it in braids and said, "Let's leave it like this until you can get it cut into a short bob." A short bob? My anxiety went out the roof. No! I'll just leave it in braids for months of chemo! I can't have cancer and my hair gone too! Please! No!

Little did I know the braids would mat and they would leave my head too! Soon all that was left was a little fluff that shed everywhere. The only good news was since my hair stopped growing the fluff had no gray roots!

No hair. No nails. No eyebrows. What was there left? Why was I being stripped of my womanliness? What had I done wrong to receive such a punishment?

I Corinthians 11:15 says a woman's long hair "is a glory to her ..." (KJV). Where is my glory, God? Why my hair? After all the time I took to grow it!

Now what? I have cancer. I am losing my pieces of me. Couldn't you spare some hair?

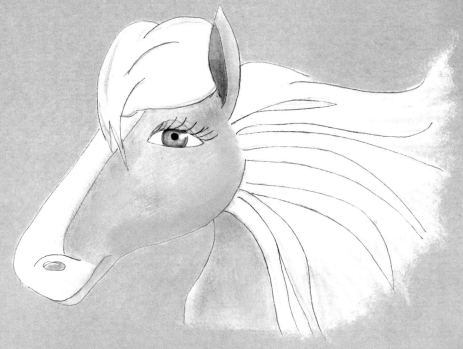

84

Luke 12:7 says: "But even the very hairs of your head are all numbered"(KJV). I am busy counting the ones falling out and wonder if God keeps track of those, too.

If I die with cancer I will die bald. Is this the way things are going to go down? Will I show up at the Pearly Gates hairless? Will Saint Peter even recognize me?

My parents? Will they even recognize me when I get there? My Dad will laugh. My Mother will cry. Where do I go from here, Oh Lord?

SHARE YOUR HAIR STORY
If you still have your hair...I'm jealous!

_____

_____

_____

_____

_____

_____

_____

What? It's Not All About the Hair?

The good news is it's not all about the hair. God still knows us bald or not. John 10:14 "I am the good shepherd and I know my sheep."

God peels away the layers. The layers of having a certain way you are supposed to look, dress, feel, and act. He, our Heavenly Father, knows how to strip us bare to the soul.

Who are we really? Who is that behind all the trimmings? Who are we at core level? Hair gone, makeup-who cares, glasses and no contacts, peeling skin, swollen face, aching joints, constant nausea... and yet God still cares for us! Amazing! When we look and feel our worst, God cares for us.

We don't have to be at our best for God to love us! He meets us where we are capable of going and wraps us in His loving arms... hair or not!

At Easter this year I had a whole new perspective of the crucifixion. For the first time I saw Jesus the man. The human body he lived in while on earth. He was stripped, literally, to the bare core for us. His mother, his family, and his friends all saw this happen. They saw Him at His worst possible physical moment dying on the cross.

He was a brave human as well as our Saviour. His dignity was destroyed, His flesh, as well as His life. You know He suffered more knowing His own mother, Mary was there.

He had no control of His circumstances and neither do we. He faced the end with patience and purpose.

Why do we suffer? Maybe there is a higher purpose in this for us, too. Being ill does make our faith stronger and we lean more on God in time of need.

HAS BEING ILL CHANGED YOUR RELATIONSHIP WITH GOD?

_____

_____

_____

_____

_____

_____

_____

_____

_____

_____

Have Faith

Have faith. We hear that phrase every day. But what is this illusive faith Jesus talked about? "Now faith is the substance of things hoped for, the evidence of things not seen" Hebrews 11:1(KJV).

Things hoped for? Does that mean our dreams and our goals? Evidence of things not seen? You can't put faith in a bottle and label it? What exactly is faith?

Faith is a heart issue. It also involves trust. "I believe in God the Father, maker of heaven and earth, and in His son Jesus Christ..." The Apostles Creed reminds us what we, as Christians, believe. If you believe you trust, hence trusting is having faith.

Are you worried about your faith wavering? We all do. It's easy to believe in a sunny day God. A God that makes the flowers bloom and our gardens grow. That is childhood faith.

As an adult it gets harder to muster up the faith when people around us start dying, we become ill and the everyday tolls of life drag us into a sinkhole of despair. Remember it doesn't take a lot of faith to get the job done!

Jesus replied, "...If ye have faith as a grain of mustard seed, ye shall say unto this mountain, Remove hence to yonder place; and it shall remove; and nothing shall be impossible unto you" Matthew 17:20 (KJV).

When I was a little girl we studied that scripture in Sunday school. I kept trying to imagine what a mustard seed looked like. Faith the size of what? I told my Mom's best friend, Katie Mae, I needed to know what a mustard seed looked like. She asked me why. I said because that is how much faith I need to have. She laughed and said she thought God would not hold me responsible or measure my faith just by the size of an elusive seed.

A couple of months later she came to my birthday party with a big smile and a tiny box. She said the answers I searched for were inside. I opened the small package to find a dainty little necklace with a small globe attached as its charm. I looked inside the globe to see an almost invisible seed.

It was a mustard seed! The thing I had searched for was right there inside my birthday present! It was so tiny I overlooked it at first. I thought it was just a dot or bubble in the surrounding glass.

That's all the faith I have to have to move a mountain? I couldn't believe it. How could that small amount of anything make such a difference? It was barely visible to the naked eye. It had no arms and legs to lift or push. It had no substance at all. How could something so miniscule and tiny make a difference?

I wore that necklace until the chain was too short to wrap around my teen age neck. I put it on every morning and asked God to give me faith. When I outgrew it I put it in my jewelry box so every time I opened the box I would be reminded how little God actually expects of us in the faith department.

Thank you Katie Mae Burch! Thank you for showing a five-year-old that the tiniest amount of faith can move a mountain! May your heavenly crown be filled with stars!

WHO INSPIRED YOU ON YOUR JOURNEY OF FAITH?
How did they help you?

_____

_____

_____

_____

HAVE YOU MOVED ANY OF YOUR OWN MOUNTAINS LATELY?

_____

_____

_____

_____

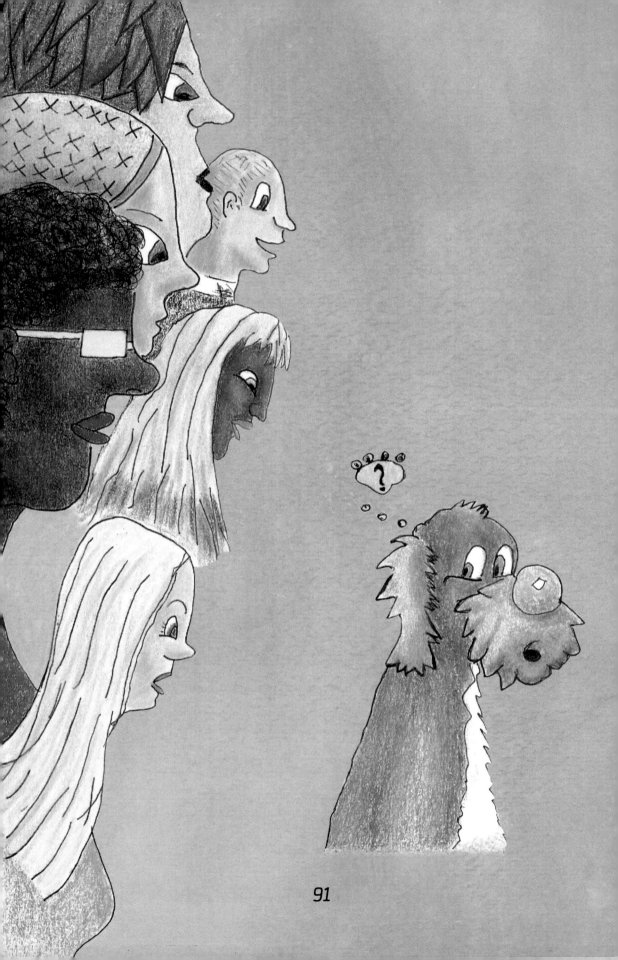

Warrior Stance, Girls!

STRESS

You are a member of a larger family unit. You feel responsible for keeping it flowing. Learn to delegate. Anyone can fold clothes and put away dishes! Think where you need help and ask for it!

If you are still on the job please, for your sake, discuss your health issue with your supervisor. Keep it brief but to the point. It's okay if you cut back to part time or take a leave of absence. Ask your body what it needs to conquer cancer.

FINANCES

Co-pays add up. Insurance doesn't cover everything. You are trying to hold your finances together as they burst at the seam. Make a budget. Downsize whatever you can. Coupon!

You may be making less yet spending more because of the illness. Hang in there. If you need to ask for help from a close family member or the church, don't be embarrassed. Everyone has their own dark night of the finances saga! Besides, when you get well you can pass that help forward to another person in need!

UNCERTAINTY

What is next? Am I going to make it through that next treatment? Will I wake up after surgery? How am I going to survive?

LOSS OF SELF

You can lose the real you easily in a long term illness. You may give up a job, social life, intimacy, and social activities. You do not have freedom to go where you want, when you want. Find the real you and don't settle for being a pin cushion! Keep laughing, it clears the air!

LOSS OF DIGNITY

So many things have been taken away from you and me. Basic things such as hair and keeping food down are gone. Our social activities may be put on pause until we get through treatments. That's okay! We can have a big party when we get well!

Push forward, Girl! You can get this Done!

Healing All Wounds

It takes time to heal a cut, scrape, or bruise. There has to be consistent daily care. This thing inside me is an invader. It is my mortal enemy. It wants to devour me whole and conquer me body and soul. It is a stranger living deep inside plotting to rule and destroy.

God tells us, "Fear thou not; for I am with thee: be not dismayed; for I am thy God: I will strengthen thee; yea, I will help thee; yea, I will uphold thee with the right hand of my righteousness" Isaiah 41:10 (KJV). No matter what we go through we have to believe He is there with us. We are not alone! Take comfort in that thought!

This cancer, this devouring fiend, is inside us and NOT those we love. It is happening to you and me, not to them. Remember they have a different perspective of your illness than you do.

Our spiritual self is also ill. We discussed this earlier. If the body is sick so is the mind, heart and soul. Think about driving down the road in a gorgeous sports car when... Cough! Out goes the transmission! Now where are you? You have a gorgeous car you can't drive!

Our bodies are still beautiful and functional. Don't forget that! We are wisely and wonderfully made! Cough! Even with our cuts, ports, baldness, and tumors we are still God's creation.

Our heart feels the bumps and reacts by sending out tears, anger, depression, self-doubt and fear. We sometimes go into a protective mode shutting down and locking up our emotions. We become numb and unfeeling. It seems easier that way.

WHAT PARTS OF YOU NEEDS HEALING TODAY?
Release! This is your safe place!

_____

_____

_____

_____

_____

Courage

I CAN DO ALL THINGS THROUGH CHRIST WHO STRENGTHENS ME

You can do this! I believe in you. You have to believe in yourself. Be strong in the Lord. Without Him how could we go thru the things we experience here on earth? Remember "I can do all things through Christ which strengthens me" Philippians 4:13 (KJV). That is my mantra. It is my daily self-talk.

You can say it when you are doing your daily chores. Say it silently. Say it out loud. Yell it to the top of your lungs in the shower. But don't scare the kids!

You CAN do this. This part of your life will be over soon. Treatment may seem like it lasts forever but that's not true. Don't feed yourself lies. You will get through this time.

This disease is a "temporary inconvenience". Take it one breath and one step at a time. My love for my family keeps me going! I visualize me here in this world with them!

I want to see my handsome son's children someday. I want to see my beautiful daughter walk down the aisle in a fairy tale wedding! Those are two of the pictures that keep me going. My love for my family. I visualize me there. Does that make sense? I see a positive picture in the future and place myself in it. If God has other plans then so be it but I am keeping positive pictures with positive goals in my mind.

Think ahead. What are some future happy pictures that involve your family and friends that you want to be in? There is room to draw. Stick figures are fine! Be sure you are IN these pictures. Enjoy!

Have Fun! Draw Away!

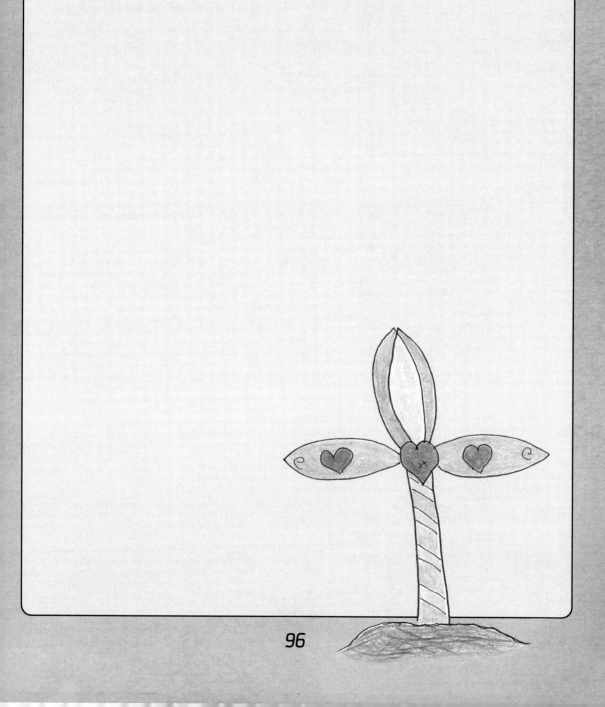

Find Your Purpose

Find something bigger than you. What would you want to leave this world, or your family, if you knew you were fixing to exit the planet?

"Jesus saith unto him, I am the way, the truth, and the life: no man cometh unto the Father, but by me" John 14:6 (KJV). Jesus left us eternal life. Through His suffering came incredible beauty and truth. You and I are still here because God has something for us to do.

I ask, "But God, couldn't I do this better WITH hair?" My family thinks I am obsessed with hair. I AM. Hence the name of the book. We laughingly pretend it doesn't matter but it does.

Crazy things happen on our way to getting well. Sometimes hair falls out, your brain fogs, and you can't stomach smells.

What do you do? Hold on and find your purpose! Why we are going through this we may never know but if we can shovel out of our own disappointments and pain maybe we can make ourselves better people. Maybe we can improve our own life or the lives of others.

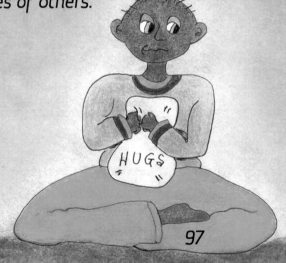

Create a goal or goals for yourself. They don't have to be big, just positive! One lady I know is knitting hats for cancer patients, one is making Welcome Bags for new people, another is drawing cards.

WHAT CAN YOU DO NOW (WITH CANCER) TO IMPROVE YOURSELF OR THE LIVES OF OTHERS AROUND YOU?

Remember you are not trying to change the world,
just finding a purpose to stay on the planet.

_____

_____

_____

_____

_____

_____

_____

Stop and Just Breathe #6

Give it ALL to God. Stop and release!

_____

_____

_____

_____

_____

_____

_____

_____

_____

_____

_____

_____

_____

_____

_____

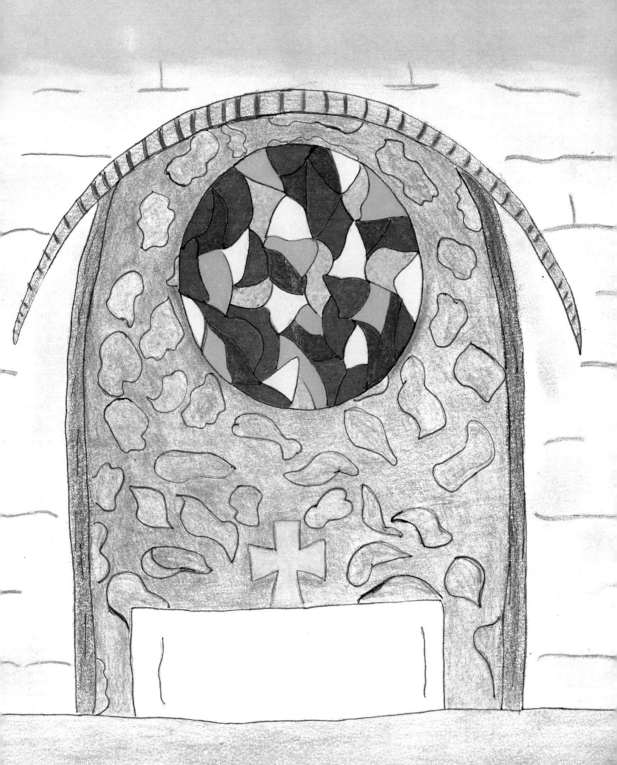

Part 7:

Angels Among Us

★☆★☆★✦★✦★✦★✦★✦★☆★✦★✦★✦★☆★✦★✦★✦

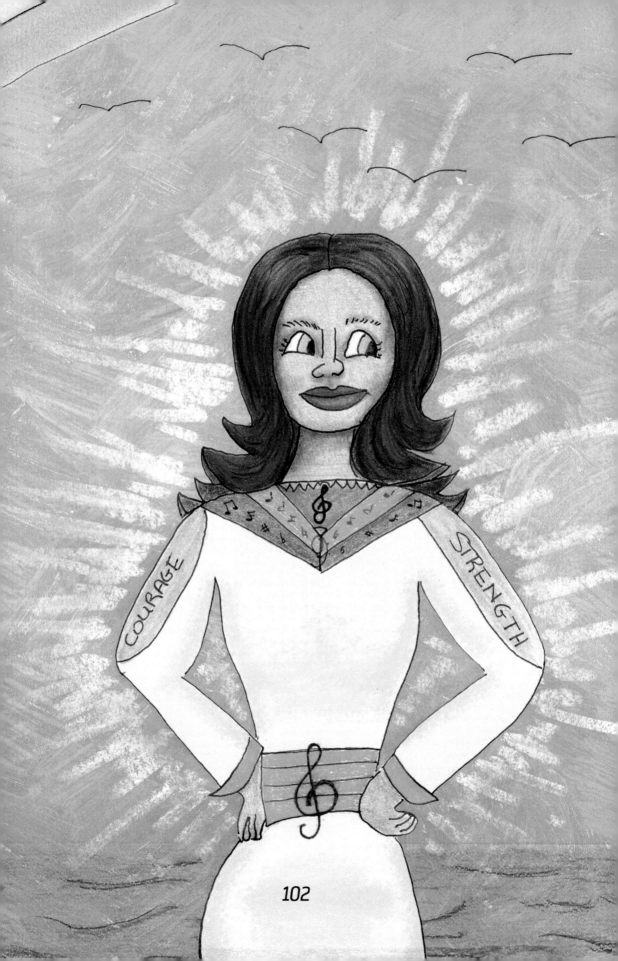

Angels Among Us

A few days after surgery, Janice and I went to the grocery store. It was going to be a short, simple first trip out to pick up coffee and oatmeal. We were reading ingredients on coffee creamers when an extremely tall woman ran by us pushing a shopping cart at an alarming rate of speed. I almost fell over! She got to the end of the aisle and looked back at us and headed straight towards us. I tried to brace myself for impact.

She stopped a few inches from me and looked me in the face and said, "Remember strength! You have to remember strength," This time she crossed her large arms and made fists across her chest. "You have to fight the enemy. Keep courage!"

Her voice was mesmerizing. All I could think of was how this woman had almost hit me and now she was telling me to be strong and have courage because it was going to be a fight. I could see her sky blue sparkling earrings swaying as she pounded her chest and then again repeated the same battle cry.

I remember saying "thank you" and giving her a weak hug. We went on to the next aisle and I never saw my angel again.

I had to ask Janice what she had just said," Strength and Courage" were the only words ringing in my ears.

Janice heard so much more! She heard:

1. Take frequent naps
2. Think of yourself and what you need
3. When people ask what they can do to help say bring over last night's leftovers I don't eat much
4. Take things slower
5. You will see things differently than you used to see them
6. Don't feel like you have to fix everyone's problems or needs
7. Take care of you
8. Have a positive attitude

These are good words to live by at any stage of our lives BUT especially now!

Own this for you and your life!!!

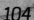

Illness brings out the best in those around you. Let your family and friends help you! You have always been in control of your own life. You did things on your own terms. Now you need a driver, a cook, a bed changer, a hug, and possibly some hair!

Fill your soul with the love they share with you. You will grow stronger with the help of your angels! Go and soar with the eagles, my friend!

Have you had an angel, from heaven or earth, appear in your life giving you a smile, a glance, time, or words of encouragement? List them here and show gratitude for their presence in your life!

SAY "THANK YOU"

_____

_____

_____

_____

_____

_____

_____

_____

_____

God is So Good!
DREAMS REALLY DO COME TRUE

In conclusion, I want to share a true joy that happened during my cancer journey! As I mentioned before, two of the things that were holding me on the planet were my kids, Amber and Alex. I wanted to see Alex as a daddy of four and Amber get married. It happened. At least one of them! I got to see my precious daughter walk down the aisle... um beach!

She and Matt, my new son, decided to move up the wedding date after my diagnosis. They made the plan to get married on the beach in the Keys. At sunset might I add? How perfect!

With this diagnosis and treatments how did I get to go? Sheer willpower and prayer!

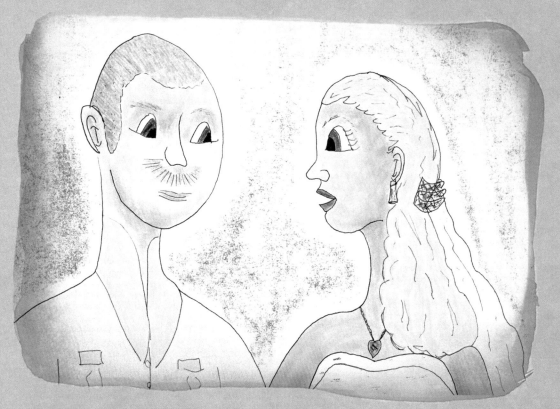

I had a severe reaction to the last treatment before the date. I had fluids three times, got a letter from my oncologist in case medical help was needed on the trip, and Alex and I boarded the plane. Two flights, three wheelchairs, and a rental car (I barfed in) later we were there!

I got to see her in all her beauty! My beloved daughter walking down the beach with the glow of love all over her face. I could see her Daddy in her golden hair and dancing eyes. I could see me in her smile.

I grieved that her Daddy was not there to see his precious baby girl get married. I celebrated that God allowed me to be there. Emotions poured! The ocean breeze blew. Amber grabbed my wig just in time so it did not become a beach relic. There was laughter, joy, gratitude.

Thank you God for keeping me on the planet to share this incredible moment of love and devotion with my family! I give You glory and praise for answered prayers. BTW Alex, no pressure on having four girls anytime soon, ha!

I believe God has given you such miracles during our time together.

WHAT ARE YOUR MIRACLES?

_____

_____

_____

_____

To Put it Mildly...
CANCER CHANGES YOU

Cancer changes you. What an understatement! We will never be the same person again. How could anyone ever be the person you were before the Big C diagnosis? Before a port was surgically implanted over your heart? Before a piece of you was removed? You had radiation burned skin? You will still be you but with a new tougher coat of paint on top of all the suffering.

You will appreciate another day alive more than most people. You will find reasons to eat that extra bite of chocolate cake. Go ahead! Swish it around in your mouth and really taste it!

Brushing that thick, luxurious hair you will grow...aaahhh! Enjoy every "it's good to have hair day"! You know you will NEVER have another bad hair day because just having hair makes even the worst hairstyle a good one!

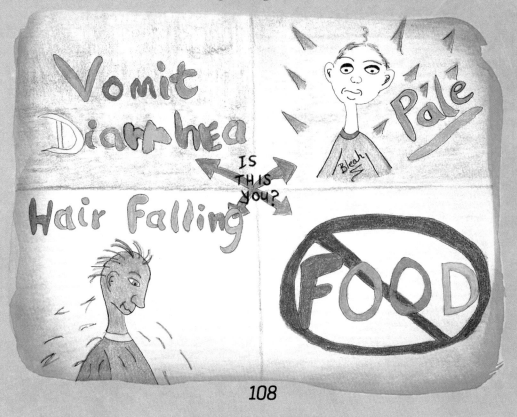

Lots of things have changed on my journey and I bet yours as well:

PRIORITIES
What is really important in this world and the next? A change of priorities changes your overall life goals and the direction your life will follow.

STRENGTH
Congratulations! You found strength you didn't know you had. Remember this strength can be carried over to other areas of your physical, mental and spiritual life.

COMPASSION
I know I am more compassionate. I can readily empathize with others going through adversity. Remember we are not alone in this life. We are a community. We need each other. Smile. Say an encouraging word. Don't forget to hug someone! You never know the secret pain in others' hearts.

FRIENDS AND FAMILY
Think back over the past months of treatments. You didn't have to do it all by yourself. You had your pack with you.

BE HONEST, REALLY HONEST
Be honest with yourself and others. Don't "sugar coat" the truth any more. You've survived this journey and so did your family. Now you know you have the strength to survive whatever the future brings. It's like wearing a t-shirt that says, "Out of my way trouble, I survived cancer, I can survive you!"

Demand respect and give it. Use your voice to stand up for your body, spirit, and soul. Continue to assert positive control over your own life and circumstances with God's help.

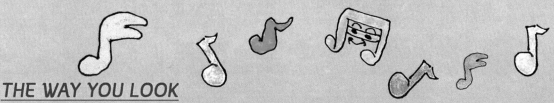

THE WAY YOU LOOK

You may look different. Not better or worse just different. You may have scars, missing body parts, a radiation tan, added wrinkles, or a new color hair. Remember you are still you! Don't forget your value and worth to God and family and friends. Most important don't forget your worth to you.

LIVE IN THE MOMENT

We live in the moment more than most people. When you have cancer your future is so uncertain you learn to appreciate each day, every event as it happens. We value them as God's gifts with the knowledge these moments are very limited.

LAUGH

Nothing relieves tension like a good laugh. Laugh, you made it to the other side of cancer. That truly deserves a thumbs up and a happy giggle!

CRY

When I was diagnosed with cancer I didn't cry in front of my kids. I thought I had to be extra brave for them. I put on a fearless front thinking I was protecting them from more pain. Inside I was screaming! Tears make us human. Remember there are no tears in heaven so let's get them all out while we are here! Share your happy AND your sad with those you love. Laughter and tears create a lasting bond between our individual souls.

ANGER

Bet you've grown a new appreciation for anger after all you have seen and been through on this journey. Remember righteous anger is a good thing!

TASTE

Is it my imagination or does everything seem different now? I don't like the same clothes, food, or activities I did before this journey started.

THANKSGIVING

Not everyone has to go into such a deep pit and claw their way out one step at a time. God believes in you and I do too. You are still here, alive, kicking, and maybe growing some hair! Understand these extra days, months, and years after treatment are the icing on the cake. Use them well and enjoy every minute!

Remember: God made only one of you, only one!

WHAT ARE SOME WAYS CANCER HAS CHANGED YOU?

I bet it has changed those around you too. How are they doing?

_____

_____

_____

_____

_____

_____

_____

_____

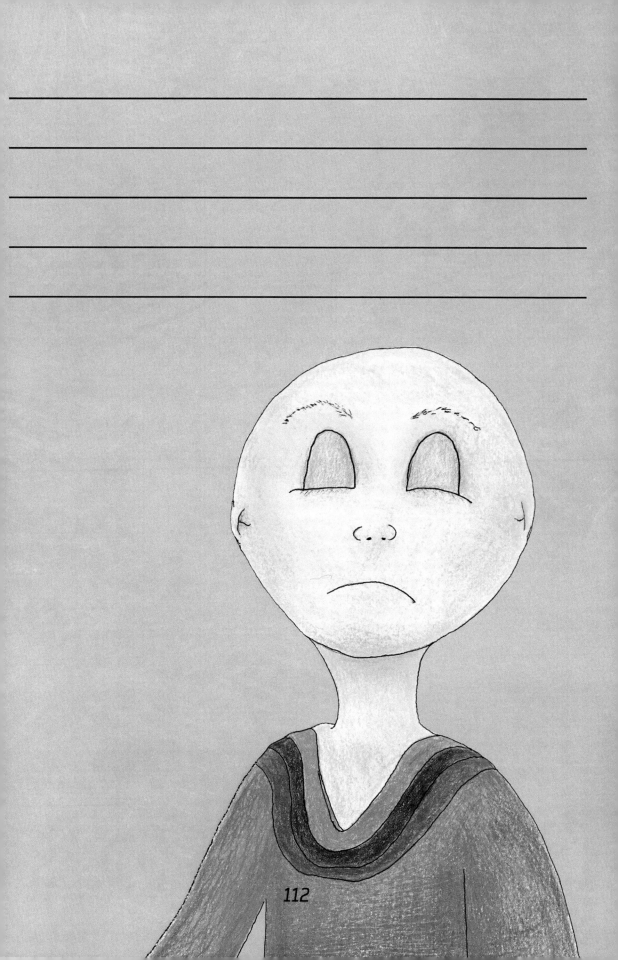

Stop and Just Breathe #7

Remember GOOD can come from our illness! Allow yourself to finally find that blessing!

God created the heavens and the earth in seven days. Our seven Stop and Release pages have hopefully enabled you to find a quiet place, a place of peace along your journey. Our lives are in the process of being recreated. Remember always, YOU are still YOU but forever changed

No matter how "woof" your diagnosis, treatments, or predicted outcome you are still a child of God. God loves you, yes you, so much!

"For God so loved the world, that he gave his only begotten Son, that whosoever believeth in him should not perish, but have everlasting life" John 3:16 (KJV).

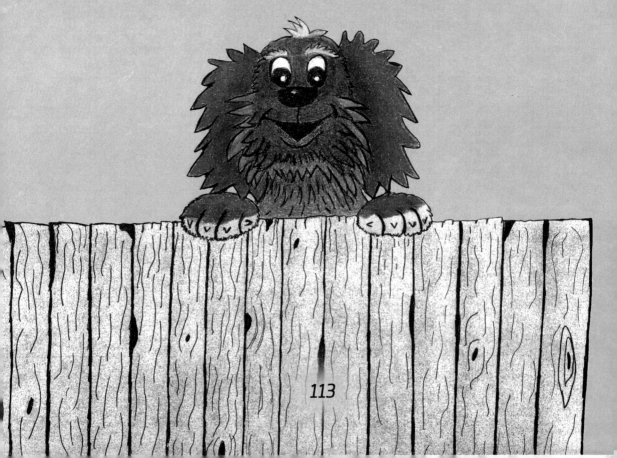

Keep that in your heart in the days and trials ahead. God gave up His Son so that you and I could be with Him forever! Take a moment to thank God for this precious gift of life!

Stop and Release.

_____

_____

_____

_____

_____

_____

_____

_____

_____

_____

_____

_____

_____

Did You Know?

Did you know that this whole book has been for and about you? As you bravely fought the Big C you also wrote your memoirs. Wow! I am so proud of you!

HOW WOULD YOU DESCRIBE YOUR TREATMENT JOURNEY?

_____

_____

_____

Okay, now for the fun stuff! Write about at least one funny thing that happened. Laughter heals and gives us joy. Remember pain and trials fade away at the end of each day but giggles last forever!

_____

_____

_____

I hope you will keep this Traveler's Guide for the rest of your life. It is a reminder of who you were and who you became. It is a legacy keepsake for you and your family. Keep it as a memoir. Better yet share your journey with others who end up on the "It's All About the Hair" journey!

REMEMBER:
You are still here because God has more for you to do!!!

It's a Wrap!

FOR NOW

Thank you for being my traveling companion on this cancer journey. It is a difficult road and knowing you are not alone is important! Scriptures tell us God is always with us. There are times I need a physical reminder of that promise.

Maybe it's considered a fleshly weakness but I need girl talk, hugs, and people around who become like "Jesus with skin on."

I hope this book has given you those hugs, humor, and a place to vent. Know you have a girlfriend who is here in the trenches with you!

When life or treatments get you down don't forget to STOP AND JUST BREATHE!

"It's All About the Hair" Book Two? Of course! We gals can't stop talking! Guess what? Next book we are going to talk about finding your way out of this disease and shoveling your way back into the world!

Whee!

See you in the next round, girlfriend!

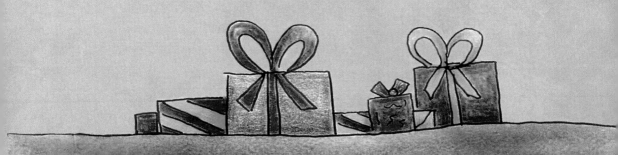

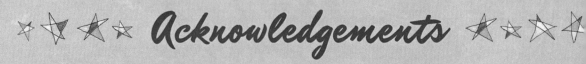

Acknowledgements

Special thanks to all the health care professionals who have guided my way through this illness. As you can tell by the length of this list it takes many skilled, compassionate individuals to take care of each patient.

Dr. Robert Creech for believing me when I said something was wrong. Thank you for getting me to the right people!

Dr. John Waples, my oncologist, a special thanks for all those early morning hospital visits when you would wake me up with a song and a smile.

Patty Stutts and Pat Brown, CCI, you always have the answers to every question and are amazing! Amanda Gambill thanks for all your scheduling expertise. Belinda McComb seeing your smile and hearing you say "Marcia, Marcia, Marcia" always brightened my day. Jillian Kinzel PA-C, Meghan Foster, PA-C, Rebecca Crawford, Emily Stevens, Tammy Wheeler, Cheryl Byers, Melissa Greer and Lindsay Sylvester thank you for your sharing your professionalism, listening and hugs.

Dr. Robert Lancaster and his surgical team at Huntsville Hospital. I so appreciate the beautiful stitches! Thanks to his office staff Dori Swaim and Liz Taylor. Great hair gals!

Dr. Beth Falkenberg, oncology radiologist, thank you for understanding with a woman's intuition. Kristin and Hannah 10:45 Monday-Friday wants to thank you for the music and for always remembering the washcloth! Thanks to Dr. Falkenburg's nurses and physician's assistant too!

Dr. Charles A. Ritchie for the numerous "almost painless" thoracentesis procedures. Twyla Pickard thanks for that beautiful smile and all the girl talk that made the procedures easier.

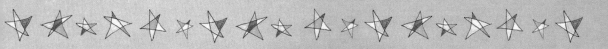

Dr Jennifer Kiessling thank you for taking care of my heart during this journey. Thank you also for listening and understanding.

Thank you to the incredible nurses and staff at Crestwood Hospital, Huntsville Hospital, Huntsville Hospital Outpatient, and physical therapists from Gentiva. A very special thanks to Renee Fabian and Laura Rutherford, my surgery recovery nurses.

Ashley B. Patterson thank you for never giving up! Nancy Johnson I always appreciate your words of wisdom.

A special thanks to Chris Reily, Lynn Anderson, and Amelia Self for their guidance and their gentle therapies.

Thanks to Jennifer Zoeller and her amazing class and book club. The origami cranes just keep flying! They will be passed on from person to person as a reminder of your kindness! Know that you will always have a special place in my heart.

Thanks to Hooks for Hope and all the beautiful caps they crochet for our hairless times. What a treat to see a basket full of new hat styles every treatment visit! It literally took away some of the sting of being there!

Thanks to Bonnie and Dave White who volunteer at CCI every Monday. Your smiles, conversations, and support are invaluable! God bless you!

Thank you Beverly D. for reading and re-reading and correcting the manuscript! Jeanne Crown thank you for sharing your life learned lessons for handling the practical aspects of a serious illness. Thanks to Betty Bates for the surgery apron and words of encouragement.

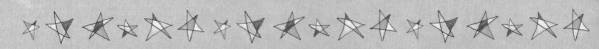

Thanks to hair stylists Rita Davis and Shelby Zimmerman for making my "little ole' bald head" feel beautiful! Your wig styling, kindness and prayers will never be forgotten. Rita, Tabetha Thompson, Stephanie Rakowski, and The Masters Salon thanks for the new fuzzy red!

My precious family Amber, Alex, and Matt who have driven me to so many appointments and had to sit by my hospital bed way too many times! Thanks to my sister-in-law Beverly who opened her home on numerous occasions for my recovery.

Thanks to Janice Parks who constantly drove the 70-mile distance between our homes. Jamie E. Logan and her sweet family shared their beach vacation with me. A week to inhale ocean air! Ah! Lynn Rea texts me every morning and night to see if I'm okay. Bonnie Duchesneau always tells me to get well or else!

Rowena Pope drove 300 miles more than once to give me hugs while I was in the hospital. Freda Austin, the queen of butterflies, has encouraged me to soar on this journey! Her awesome son Billy is a survivor!

Thanks to Suzanne Viars for encouraging words! To all the members of the Sandra J. Bryant Bosom Buddies Breast Cancer Support Group at CCI a word of appreciation. The fashion show was an amazing, healing experience!

Virginia and Chris Reily thank you for the beautiful dress, jewelry and fabulous lipstick! Your kindness and generosity melted my heart!

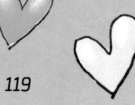

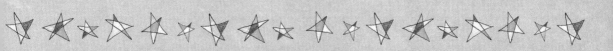

Thanks to Marcia Jones, Maria Martinez, Jo Williams, and Marilena Harris for being present on this journey. St. John the Baptist Church I cherish the beautiful prayer blanket you crocheted and had blest. Thanks for all the prayers at Mass and in the classroom. I felt them.

Jacob Fairchild thank you for the amazing cover design. Nathan Massengill I appreciate your support and artistic guidance. Kevin Stokes thanks for showing me how to draw hands. Xia Blanche thanks for scanning and encouragement.. Mandi Cook you are a true blessing and a gift from God!

Heavenly thanks to Michelle Putman. We met in a wig store, of course! She chose the blonde. I chose the redhead! Thank you for sharing the journey with me!

My dear friend, Mary Drake was a few years ahead of me in the fight and always had a positive attitude and a healing prayer. I miss her and feel her angel prayers every day!

I am grateful for all the healing prayers and encouraging words from all my family, friends, the girl squad, fellow colleagues, students and church family. Words cannot express my gratitude. Thank you! Thank you! I love you! I could not have walked this journey without you!

Gratitude to God for every new day on the planet!

PS. - Congratulations!
CONGRATULATIONS YOU HAVE BEEN CHOSEN!

Remember how our elementary teachers gave us stickers and badges? Gee, what an honor to be chosen Student of the Week, line leader, and book collector! Did you practice and practice piano so you could get to the certificate at the end of the book?

Well, why should children have all the fun? Let's join in! Why? Because it's your turn to receive the "bestest" award!

Use the enclosed certificate

OR:

Make this a really, really big project and add poster board, construction paper, and of course lots and lots of glitter, girlfriend! Let's go all out here!!!

How about having an IT'S ALL ABOUT THE HAIR autograph party to create your special awards? Your family members and friends can receive awards for being such an incredible support team through this journey!

REMEMBER THERE IS NOTHING PRETTY OR GLAMOUROUS ABOUT CANCER BUT YOU!!!!!

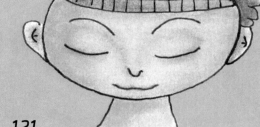

Certificate

IN YOUR HONOR

_____ has been chosen for the "It's All About the Hair" Award.

YOUR NAME

You have proven to yourself and to those around you what an incredible and courageous gal you are! You are a shining star and a true blessing from God!

Congratulations!

Marcia Ashford

Have friends & family sign too!

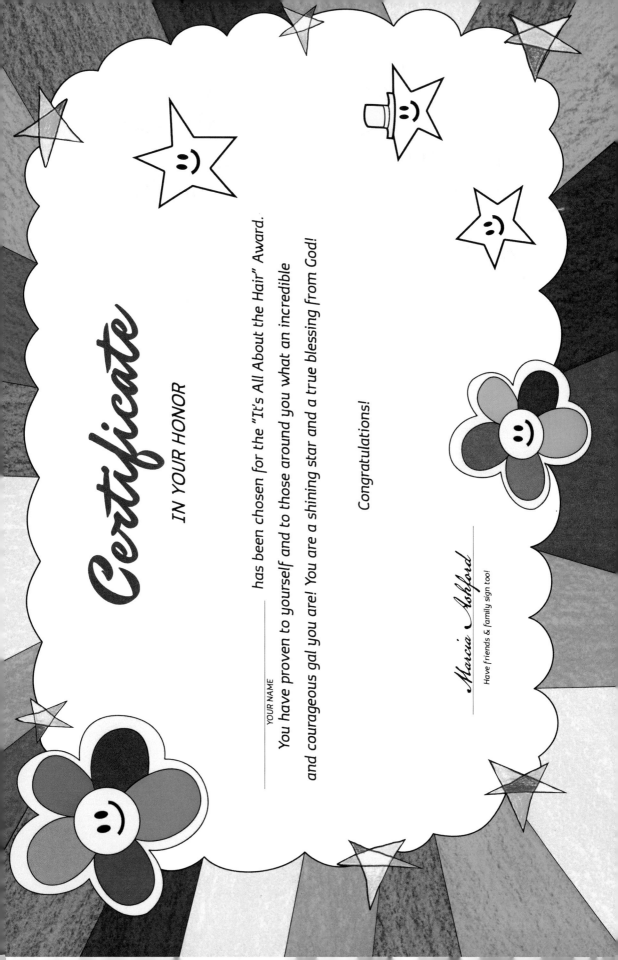

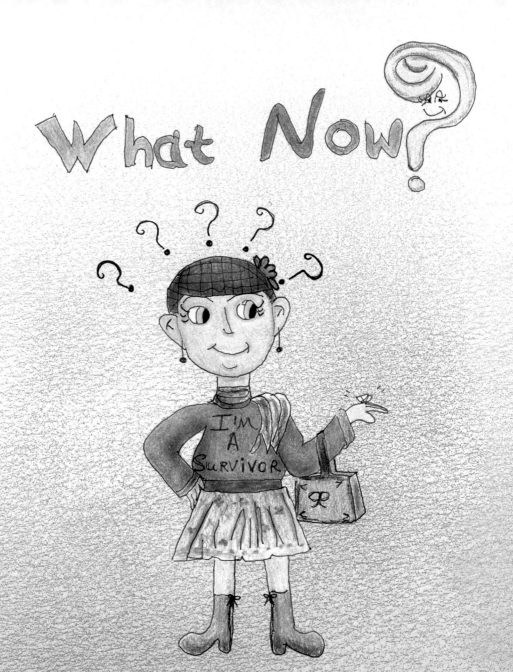

What Now?

"It's All About the Hair Two"
Coming SOON!

www.marciaashford.com

Made in United States
North Haven, CT
21 April 2022

18459416R00073